Food Facts at a Glance

Food Facts at a Glance

A Quick Reference Guide for Choosing

Wholesome, Nutritious Foods

Ginger Grant

GG Publications, Ann Arbor, MI

Visit our Web site: foodfactsataglance.com

ISBN: 978-0-615-41174-3

Library of Congress Control Number: 2010915582
(Catalog-in-Publication Data pending)

Published by GG Publications, Ann Arbor, Michigan
Book design by Paula Newcomb

Contents

Introduction

Do you want to eat better? Do you want to improve your family's diet? Most of us do.

And it's not surprising most of us want to eat better, or at least think we should. Every day there's another article in the media about how our diets are ruining our health.

"You need at least five servings of vegetables a day."

"You should give your family more fresh food—cut down on processed food."

"Everyone eats too much fat."   "Everyone eats too many carbs."

"Eat local."   "Eat colorful foods."

Healthy eating—it's an admirable goal. And there's no shortage of information out there to help you achieve it. But the information comes to us haphazardly, unpredictably. It's often buried in books with so much information that we don't have time to sort through all the words to find what we need. Or, we see interesting facts in a magazine article at the doctor's office, and then promptly forget where we saw it and what it said.

Food Facts At A Glance is your answer. Here is information on healthy foods, nutrition, and dieting in list format and short topics, easy to access, quick and to the point. It's every list you ever wanted to keep, or every article clipped and then misplaced, or every bit of information you wish you could remember—all in one basic reference book.

Maybe you want to know why you should choose whole grain bread over white bread. Or maybe one of your kids is lobbying for French fries, and you'd like to find a tempting alternative.

In this book you can find:
- answers to questions that come up daily about how to exchange fresh, whole foods for processed foods;
- complete information about vitamins and minerals in easy-to-read table format—how much you need and where to get it;

- simple explanations of concepts found in popular media—like your BMI, the glycemic index, omega 3's—in just a few short sentences.

Every time I read an article about the benefits of fresh vegetables and unprocessed grains—antioxidants, vitamins and minerals, fiber—I vow to improve my diet. I promise myself I will cook more and eat less take out; I'll go to the local farmers market every weekend; and I'll buy organic beans and grains in bulk from the food coop. But I get busy and quickly forget my vows.

Every time I see a list outlining the best sources of vitamins, of fiber, of critical minerals, I either clip it, or note where I saw it. I file it away so I can reference it when necessary. But I never do. I forget where I put it. Or I'm not at my desk when the questions come up. Or I get too busy to clip it and then forget where I saw it.

All that information is collected here in *Food Facts At A Glance* —in one small volume you can keep nearby and quickly flip to the page you need.

Most of us choose what to eat several times a day. For something so common and so compelling, surprisingly few of us know much about food—what it's made of, how it's grown, and how it functions in our bodies. In a way, that is an excellent state of affairs, because if we had to learn all there is to know about growing food, about our nutritional needs, and about metabolic functions, many of us might starve.

If food were harder to come by, we'd probably pay more attention to food's nutrient value and how long each food keeps us from getting hungry again. But with an abundance of affordable, appealing food so readily available, we are free to pick and choose foods that provide other benefits besides satisfying hunger. There's nothing wrong with that. Eating has many legitimate benefits, including pleasure and social interactions, and most of us in the developed world are lucky to enjoy all the delights foods have to offer.

In spite of this variety and abundance, many of us have become more and more interested in altering our food choices in favor of improving our health and avoiding illness, or slowing the aging process by avoiding overly processed foods. *Food Facts At A Glance* is the place to start. In this book you'll find all the information you need to make healthy food choices.

You won't find any *shoulds* or *musts* in this book. What you will find is easy-to-access information that will help you decide what foods to try, what recipes to experiment with. *Food Facts At A Glance* isn't about what will work, what is best for you, what you should do to be healthy. You are the best judge of that. But you need information to make those judgments.

Food Facts At A Glance is full of useful information presented succinctly, without any opinions or prescriptions. Our bodies handle food very differently. Different strategies for weight control work for different people. Food preferences vary. Family situations change. Busy people need information when they need it, in a format that guarantees you can find what you need in the shortest time possible.

How to Use *Food Facts at a Glance*

Check out the Table of Contents to get an overview of how the information is organized—the first section is on food—what it's made of and where all the vitamins and minerals are. The second section is on cooking and eating. The third section provides dozens of tips for preparing healthy meals, and the fourth is all about staying healthy. You can find the information that interests you the most, and skim through all the lists and short topics in that section.

Or, the extensive, cross-referenced index allows you to look up a specific food, or nutrient, or topic, and find all the pages with relevant information.

You may even find some of the lists so interesting that you'll want to skim through them, knowing you can easily get back to a particular fact. The information is presented in short lists or brief explanations, so you can dip into the book whenever you have a minute or two to spare.

I have carefully studied dozens of books and websites on food and nutrition, so you don't have to. The information in *Food Facts At A Glance* comes from that research, as well as from years of experience thinking and reading about food and eating patterns, managing a life-long weight problem, dealing with diabetes that has plagued most of the members of my family for years, and cooking my way through many diet cookbooks.

The facts in *Food Facts At A Glance* come primarily from research conducted and reported by the USDA—the U.S. Department of Agriculture—which is responsible for protecting our food supply. The USDA maintains an extensive website of information on food, with a powerful search capacity by which you can look up the nutrient profiles for thousands of foods, even many highly processed and prepared foods like frozen and boxed entrees, cereals, and breads. (See usda.gov) Other sources include well-respected medical reference books, textbooks, and some popular books on nutrition and dieting. The bibliography lists all relevant sources, including a list of my favorite writers.

While I have tried hard to check and recheck the accuracy of the nutrient data, there is bound to be variation from other published sources. This is due to variations in how food is grown, including variations in soil and rainfall, how food is harvested, how long it takes from harvesting to retail stores, how it is stored, and how processed foods are manufactured. Further, there are variations in measuring and testing processes in different labs. And, the reporting of nutrient values varies by the weight, volume, and serving sizes of foods assessed.

A personal note:

Food Facts At A Glance is a collection of information you can use to decide for yourself what to eat. Some people do well with specific directions, with rules about what to eat and what not to eat. I am not one of them. I like to find someone who knows more than I, or read a guidebook for ideas, and then use what I learn from them to find my own way. *Food Facts At A Glance* can help.

The reason I personally don't like "shoulds" is because I have learned from experience that what scientists and physicians know *for sure* about how our bodies handle food is slim and iffy at best, and evolves over time. Digestion and nutrient metabolism are very complicated, with a multitude of pathways and processes that are very hard to untangle. Articles in the popular media reporting scientific study results are often full of unwarranted interpretations. It is always good to be skeptical.

"What Should I Eat?" is easy. Eat any food that appeals to you. Eat anything you want. There is no bad food. All food serves some useful benefit. Even foods with so-called "empty calories," are not bad choices, because most of them provide enormous pleasure, which is as legitimate a reason for eating as hunger and health. Ice cream, anyone?

The "why" of eating is also easy. We choose to eat for many different reasons: hunger, nutritional needs, social participation, peer pressure, mood management, and pleasure seeking. All of these "whys" are reasonable, and serve different purposes for each of us.

My philosophy for healthy eating is:

1. learn all that interests you about food and nutrition—could be a lot or only a little;
2. experiment with what works for you; try various foods and recipes,
3. then use what you learn to decide the kind of eating plan you want to follow;
4. and remember, once you have a general plan in mind, rules are made to be broken.
5. Everything in moderation, including moderation. Somebody said that. I wish it had been me.

PART 1

Food and Nutrition Basics

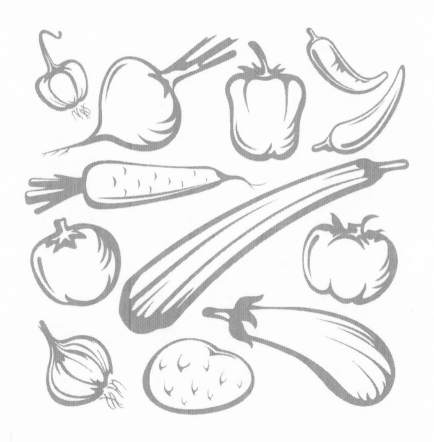

1 Essentials At A Glance

- Here is a quick look at what we need in our diets every day, or at least most days, in order to stay healthy and happy.
- The government has established these dietary recommendations (RDA's or AI's*) for protein and 18 essential vitamins and minerals. The reason carbohydrates, fats, and other trace minerals are not included in the list is that it is assumed we get enough of these no matter what we eat.
- (See "Vitamins—What We Need Where to Get Them," and "Minerals—What We Need and Where to Get Them," for more detailed information.)

NUTRIENT	MALE	FEMALE	BEST SOURCES
Protein	52 g	45 g	Lean meat, fish, nuts, beans
Vitamin A	900 re/ 2,970 IU**	700 re/ 2,310 IU**	Orange and yellow vegetables
Vitamin C	90 mg	75 mg	Citrus fruits, peppers, broccoli
Vitamin D	5 mcg/ 200 iu	5 mcg/ 200 iu	Sunlight, fish, eggs
Vitamin E	15 a-te (mg)	15 a-te (mg)	Nuts and seeds, shellfish
Vitamin K	120 mcg***	90 mcg***	Cruciferous & dark green vegetables
Thiamin (B1)	1.2 mg	1.1 mg	Peas, beans, leafy greens, pork, fish
Riboflavin (B2)	1.3 mg	1.1 mg	Beans, nuts, dairy, lean meat, eggs
Niacin (B3)	16 ne (mg)	14 ne (mg)	Beans, peas, nuts, lean meat, fish
Vitamin B6	1.3 mg	1.3 mg	Legumes, potatoes, lean meat, fish
Folate (B9)	400 mcg	400 mcg	Dark green vegetables, corn, beans
Vitamin B12	2.4 mcg	2.4 mcg	Fish, lean meat, dairy, eggs
Calcium	1,000 mg	1,000 mg	Dairy, almonds, leafy greens
Phosphorus	700 mg	700 mg	Lean meat, eggs, whole grains
Magnesium	420 mg	320 mg	Whole grains, dairy, nuts, beans
Iron	8 mg	15 mg	Lean meat, oysters, whole grains
Zinc	11 mg	8 mg	Oysters, lean meat, beans, nuts
Copper	900 mcg	900 mcg	Oysters, nuts, potatoes, grains
Iodine	150 mcg	150 mcg	Added to table salt
Selenium	70 mcg	55 mcg	Lean meat, Brazil nuts, whole grains
Fiber	35 g	25 g	Unprocessed vegetables, fruits, grains, and nuts

*The familiar RDA (Recommended Daily Allowance) has been changed to AI (Adequate Intake)
**RE=Retinol Equivalents; IU-International Units. Vitamin manufacturers use both designations
***Note that some vitamin amounts are in mg (milligrams) and some in mcg (micrograms); a gram is 1000 milligrams, and a milligram is 1000 micrograms.

NUTRIENT	MALE	FEMALE	BEST SOURCES
Carbohydrate	180 g	150 g	Unprocessed vegetables, fruits, and grains
Fat	45 g	35 g	Vegetable oils, fish, meat, eggs

Note: You can find complete nutrient profiles on every food using the search function at www.usda.gov

Essentials for Children

- Kids are not just miniature adults. Not only are they smaller, but their bodily functions are still developing, so they metabolize vitamins and minerals differently than adults.
- Generally, children need less of everything, and their needs change as they grow.
- Rapid development of tissues like bone, muscle, and skin mean that kids especially need adequate B12, vitamin K, and calcium.

RDA OR AI*	INFANT TO 6 MONTHS	6–12 MONTHS	1–3 YEARS	4–8 YEARS	8–13 YEARS
Vitamin A IU	1,875	1,875	2,000	2,500	3,500
Vitamin C (mg)	*	*	15	25	45
Vitamin D (mcg)	5	5	5	5	5
Vitamin E IU	9	9	9	10	16
Vitamin K (mcg)	5	10	15	20	30
Thiamin (B1 mg)	0.2	0.3	0.5	0.6	0.9
Riboflavin (B2 (mg)	0.3	0.4	0.5	0.6	0.9
Niacin (B3) (mg)	2.0	3.0	6.0	8.0	12.0
Vitamin B6 (mg)	0.1	0.3	0.5	0.6	1.0
Folate (Bb9) (mcg)	65	80	150	200	300
Vitamin B12 (mcg)	0.4	0.5	0.9	1.2	1.8
Calcium (mg)	210	270	500	800	1,300
Phosphorus (mg)	200	300	500	800	1,300
Magnesium (mg)	30	75	80	130	240
Iron (mg)	6	10	10	10	11
Zinc (mg)	5	5	10	10	10
Copper (mg)	0.4–0.6	0.6–0.7	0.7–1.0	1.0–1.5	1.0–2.0
Iodine (mcg)	40	50	70	90	120
Selenium (mcg)	15	20	20	30	40

* RDA = Recommended Daily Allowance
* AI = Adequate Intake
Source: www.usda.gov

Essentials for Older Adults

- As people age, bodily functions change as well. Nerves communicate slightly more slowly, decreasing reaction times; muscles react more slowly.
- Digestion, absorption and metabolic rates also decrease, lowering the need for calories. With fewer calories comes less intake of vitamins and minerals.
- Generally, older adults need more B vitamins, especially choline and B12.
- Calcium needs are even more important, due to losses in bone density. Vitamin D intake could become inadequate because older adults are not outdoors as much as their younger friends.
- Due to a slowing of digestive processes, seniors should concentrate on getting plenty of fiber.

RDA OR AI* AGES 51–70	MALE	FEMALE	TOLERABLE UI** AGES 51–70	MALE	FEMALE
Vitamin A (mcg)	900	700	Vitamin A (mcg)	3,000	3,000
Vitamin C (mg)	90	75	Vitamin C (mg)	2,000	2,000
Vitamin D (mcg)	15	15	Vitamin D (mcg)	50	50
Vitamin E (mg)	15	15	Vitamin E (mg)	1,000	1,000
Vitamin K (mcg)	120	90	Vitamin K (mcg)	ND	ND
Thiamin (B1 mg)	1.2	1.1	Thiamin (B1 mg)	ND	ND
Riboflavin (B2 (mg)	1.3	1.1	Riboflavin (B2 (mg)	ND	ND
Niacin (B3) (mg)	16	14	Niacin (B3) (mg)	35	35
Vitamin B6 (mg)	1.7	1.5	Vitamin B6 (mg)	100	100
Folate (B9) (mcg)	400	400	Folate (B9) (mcg)	1,000	1,000
Vitamin B12 (mcg)	2.4	2.4	Vitamin B12 (mcg)	ND	ND
Biotin (mg)	30	30	Biotin (mg)	ND	ND
Choline (mg)	550	425	Choline (mg)	3,500	3,500
Calcium (mg)	1,200	1,200	Calcium (mg)	2,500	2,500
Magnesium (mg)	420	320	Magnesium (mg)	350	350
Sodium (mg)	1,300	1,300	Sodium (mg)	2,300	2,300
Potassium (mg)	4,700	4,700	Potassium (mg)	ND***	ND
Iron (mg)	8	8	Iron (mg)	45	45
Copper (mg)	9	9	Copper (mg)	100	100
Zinc (mg)	11	8	Zinc (mg)	40	40
Iodine (mcg)	150	150	Iodine (mcg)	1,100	1,100

* RDA = Recommended Daily Allowance
* AI = Adequate Intake
** UI = International units
*** ND = Values not determined
Source: www.usda.gov

RDA OR AI* AGES 70+	MALE	FEMALE	TOLERABLE UI* AGES 70+	MALE	FEMALE
Vitamin A (mcg)	900	700	Vitamin A (mcg)	3,000	3,000
Vitamin C (mg)	90	75	Vitamin C (mg)	2,000	2,000
Vitamin D (mcg)	15	15	Vitamin D (mcg)	50	50
Vitamin E (mg)	15	15	Vitamin E (mg)	1,000	1,000
Vitamin K (mcg)	120	90	Vitamin K (mcg)	ND	ND
Thiamin (B1 mg)	1.2	1.1	Thiamin (B1 mg)	ND	ND
Riboflavin (B2 (mg)	1.3	1.1	Riboflavin (B2 (mg)	ND	ND
Niacin (B3) (mg)	16	14	Niacin (B3) (mg)	35	35
Vitamin B6 (mg)	1.7	1.5	Vitamin B6 (mg)	100	100
Folate (B9) (mcg)	400	400	Folate (B9) (mcg)	1,000	1,000
Vitamin B12 (mcg)	2.4	2.4	Vitamin B12 (mcg)	ND	ND
Biotin (mg)	30	30	Biotin (mg)	ND	ND
Choline (mg)	550	425	Choline (mg)	3,500	3,500
Calcium (mg)	1,200	1,200	Calcium (mg)	2,500	2,500
Magnesium (mg)	420	320	Magnesium (mg)	350	350
Sodium (mg)	1,200	1,200	Sodium (mg)	2,300	2,300
Potassium (mg)	4,700	4,700	Potassium (mg)	ND	ND
Iron (mg)	8	8	Iron (mg)	45	45
Copper (mg)	9	9	Copper (mg)	100	100
Zinc (mg)	11	8	Zinc (mg)	40	40
Iodine (mcg)	150	150	Iodine (mcg)	1,100	1,100

* RDA = Recommended Daily Allowance
  AI = Adequate Intake
  UI = Upper Intake Level
  ND = Values not determined
Source: www.usda.gov

2 Number of Servings Per Day
Another Way to Look at Dietary Essentials

1. Aim for **balance** between food groups; no proportion is the right proportion.
2. If it all seems too complicated, go for **equal calories** of protein, fat, and carbohydrate. Just remember that proteins and carbs have about 4 calories per gram, and fat has roughly twice that (9 calories per gram).
3. Try to eat fruits and vegetables of **many colors**, so you cover all the vitamins and minerals.
4. Everything in **moderation**, including moderation!

Recommended Number of Servings Per Day
(by calorie intake)

FOOD GROUP	1600 CALS inactive women and elderly	2,200 CALS most children active women and men	2,800 CALS teenagers and very active adults	WHAT IS A SERVING?
Breads, crackers,* cakes, & cookies	3	6	7	1 slice bread or cake 4 crackers, 2 cookies, 1/2 bagel
Cereals*	1	1.5	1.5	1/2 cup dry or cooked hot cereal
Rice, pasta*	1	2	2	1/2 cup cooked
Vegetables— leafy or watery	3	4	4	1 cup, 1/2 cup chopped
Vegetables— starchy	1	1.5	2	1/2 cup cooked
Fruit	2	3	4	1 med. raw, 1/2 cup cooked 3/4 cup juice
Milk products (milk, yogurt)	2.5	2.5	2.5	1 cup 1/2 cup cottage/ricotta cheese
Meat, fish, beans	2	3	4	3 oz. meat or fish 1/2 cup beans

FOOD GROUP	1600 CALS inactive women and elderly	2,200 CALS most children active women and men	2,800 CALS teenagers and very active adults	WHAT IS A SERVING?
Cheese, butter	1	1	2	1.5 oz.
Eggs	1	1	1	1 egg (1 oz.)
Nuts	1	1	1	1/2 cup, 2 tbsp peanut butter
Fats, oil	1	1	2	2 tbsp

*try to make at least 1/2 of these servings whole grain

Note: These amounts are very approximate and can be spread over more than one day.

3 What Foods Are Made of
Carbohydrates, Proteins, and Fats

Carbohydrates

- Carbohydrates are compounds in our food that are converted to sugars (glucose) by the body during digestion and metabolism.
- Glucose is the fuel our bodies turn into energy. Most of our glucose is ferried by the blood to the cells in our tissues, where it is converted to energy; a small amount remains in the liver as a ready supply for brain and nerve cells. A small amount of glucose is needed to build cartilage and bone. Excess glucose is converted to fat and stored in fat cells.

(see "Chapter 27—Glycemic Index and Glycemic Load" for more information on carbs.

UNPROCESSED & MINIMALLY PROCESSED CARBS	MANUFACTURED (PROCESSED) CARBS
Sugars (sugar, honey, molasses, etc.)	Canned, bottled, and dried fruits
Fruits	Canned and bottled veggies
Vegetables	Fruit and vegetable juices
Grains	Breads and cereals
Legumes (beans, peas, lentils)	Snacks (crackers, chips, etc.)
Milk products	Cakes, cookies, & pastries
Nuts & seeds (carbs, protein, and fat)	Other sweets (jello, puddings, soda, powdered drinks, candy)

Proteins

- Proteins are compounds in animals and plants that help the body perform every one of its functions, give cells their structure, and facilitate cell growth, repair and maintenance.
- Dietary proteins are metabolized into amino acids and peptides, which are used to make proteins in our bodies. The body cannot store protein; excess protein is burned for energy or converted to fat by the body.

UNPROCESSED & MINIMALLY PROCESSED PROTEINS	MANUFACTURED (PROCESSED) PROTEINS
Milk products (milk, cottage cheese, farmers cheese, yogurt and ice cream)	Processed & canned meats & fish
Nuts & seeds	Frozen, canned, & boxed entrees
Meat, fish, and eggs	Tofu and tempeh (soybeans)
Cheeses	Trail mix & granola/protein bars
Legumes (beans, peas, lentils)	

Fats

- Fats are substances in food which our bodies convert to fatty acids through metabolism.
- Fats are used by the body to form cell membranes, and can also be burned for energy.
- Visceral fat cushions internal organs and shields nerve and brain cells.
- Fat under the skin provides insulation.
- Excess fat is stored in fat cells throughout the body.

(See "Chapter 10—All About Fats" for more information on fats).

UNPROCESSED & MINIMALLY PROCESSED FATS	MANUFACTURED (PROCESSED) FATS
Milk products	Processed & canned meats & fish
Nuts & seeds	Frozen, canned, & boxed entrees
Meat, fish, and eggs	Snacks (crackers, chips, etc)
Cheeses, butter, and cream	Trail mix & granola/protein bars
	Cakes, cookies, and pastries
	Nut and seed oils, spreads, and dressings

Combination foods

- Some foods have two types of nutrients in significant amounts, sometimes in a pretty even balance.
- Only two types of foods have all three food groups in significant amounts:
  - nuts and seeds, and
  - milk products (milk, cottage cheese, farmers cheese, yogurt, and ice cream).

UNPROCESSED & MINIMALLY PROCESSED FOODS

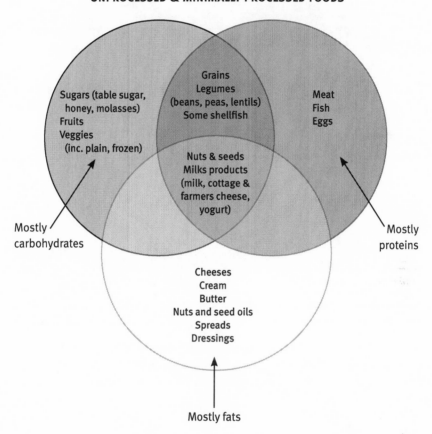

MANUFACTURED (PROCESSED) FOODS

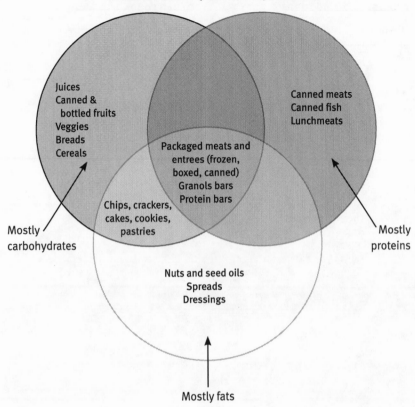

Juices
Canned &
 bottled fruits
Veggies
Breads
Cereals

Canned meats
Canned fish
Lunchmeats

Packaged meats and
entrees (frozen,
boxed, canned)
Granols bars
Protein bars

Chips, crackers,
cakes, cookies,
pastries

Mostly
carbohydrates

Mostly
proteins

Nuts and seed oils
Spreads
Dressings

Mostly fats

4 Carbohydrates, Proteins, and Fats
How Much of Each?

There is little or no consensus among nutritionists and fitness gurus regarding optimal proportion of dietary carbohydrates, proteins, and fats, nor has there been much research done on the topic. What research does seem to suggest is that bodies vary so significantly in the ways they digest, absorb, and metabolize nutrients that the best answer is the proportion that succeeds in maintaining a healthy weight.

There is general agreement that the following proportions are reasonable:

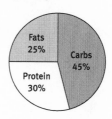

Recommended Number of Servings

How do nutritionists come up with the recommended number of servings of each food group per day? They divide the number of calories needed for each food group by number of calories in a gram; then divide the number of grams needed each day by the number of grams in an average serving. There you have it! The average number of servings you need per day. Here's an illustration:

NUMBER OF CALORIES OF EACH NEEDED PER DAY:	1200 KCALS	1500 KCALS	2000 KCALS
Carbohydrates — 35–45%	420–540	525–675	700–900
Proteins — 25–35%	300–420	375–525	500–700
Fats — 15–25%	180–300	225–375	300–500

which would require approximately (number of grams for each):

	1200 KCALS	1500 KCALS	2000 KCALS
Carbohydrates (1 g = 4 calories)	105–135 g	132–168 g	175–225 g
Proteins (1g = 4 calories)	75–105 g	94–130 g	125–175 g
Fats 1 g = 9 calories)	20–33 g	25–42 g	33–56 g

Recommended serving size:

Carbohydrates: ½ cup, about 15 grams or 60–80 calories
   (depending on density)
Proteins: about 3 oz., 25 grams or 100 calories
Fats: about 1 Tbsp, or 1 oz., about 12 grams, 100 calories.

Note: Pay attention to how small the serving sizes are compared to how you normally eat. The number of serving sizes, especially of carbohydrates may seem high, but it is because the serving size is small.

Average serving size divided by number of grams required each day equals approximately:

	SERVINGS FOR 1200 KCALS	SERVINGS FOR 1500 KCALS	SERVINGS FOR 2000 KCALS
Carbohydrates	7–9	9–11	12–15
Proteins	3–4	4–5	5–7
Fats	2–3	2–3	3–5

5 Vitamins
How Much We Need & Where To Get Them

- Vitamins are chemical compounds that help our bodies—our organs and hormones and enzymes — do their jobs.
- We get vitamins in two ways:
  - We ingest them in the foods we eat
  - They are made in our bodies by our organs, other compounds, and sometimes even by bacteria
- The amount we need varies considerably between vitamins (see chart)
- Some vitamins (A, D, E, and K) are *fat soluble,* which means they can be stored in our organs and tissues and can build up in our bodies. For this reason, if you take supplements, it is important to monitor how much you are getting from your food and how much from supplements, so you don't get too much.
- Other vitamins (all the B vitamins and Vitamin C) are *water soluble.* They are easily flushed out of our bodies. For this reason, it is unlikely you would ingest too much.
- Most vitamins occur in both plant and animal food sources, be-cause animals eat plants and the vitamins end up in their tissues. But there are some exceptions:
  - Folic acid (vitamin B9) is found predominantly in plants;
  - Cobalimin (vitamin B12) is found only in animal products (though many grain products are fortified with vitamin B12);
  - Ascorbic acid (vitamin C) is found only in plants, especially citrus fruit;
  - Calciferol (vitamin D) is found mostly in animal food sources (though many grain products are fortified with vitamin D)
- Certain compounds act like vitamins and are called vitamins (choline, inositol, PABA); some nutritionists do not consider them vitamins because our bodies readily manufacture them.
- Most nutritionists and health care providers believe we should get our vitamins from the foods we eat, and that people who eat enough calories and a variety of foods should have no problem getting sufficient amounts. However, most also agree with those who choose to take a multivitamin supplement, knowing that

some of us do not get sufficient variety in our diets to be sure we are getting sufficient amounts of every necessary nutrient.

Below is a list of all the vitamins we need, including those that are made by our bodies. Compare this list with the list on your multivitamin supplement to make sure the formula is right for you.

VITAMIN	NAME	BEST PLANT SOURCES	BEST ANIMAL SOURCES	ADULT RDA/AI* WOMEN
A Beta Carotene** (fat soluble)	Retinol	• Sweet potato • Carrots • Winter squash (acorn, butternut, etc) • Spinach • Apricots	• Chicken or beef liver • Milk • Eggs • Fish • Butter	70 mcg 2,333 IU
B1 (water soluble)	Thiamin	• Oranges • Peas • Peanut butter • Wheat germ • Beans • Whole grains	• Pork • Liver • Fish	1.1 mg
B2 (water soluble)	Riboflavin	• Beans • Nuts • Leafy green vegetables • Avocados • Mushrooms	• Milk • Dairy products • Meat • Mackerel	1.3 mg
B3 (water soluble)	Niacin	• Beans • Peas • Peanut butter • Nuts • Mushrooms • Asparagus	• Lamb • Chicken • Fish, esp. tuna, salmon • Milk • Dairy products	14 mg
B5 (water soluble)	Pantothenic acid	• Whole grains • Beans, lentils • Peas • Mushrooms • Broccoli	• Liver • Meat • Fish • Chicken • Egg yolks • Milk	5 mg

ADULT RDA/AI* MEN	IMPORTANT FOR:	VITAMINS AND MINERALS THAT HELP ABSORPTION	DAILY UPPER LIMIT
90 mcg 3,000 iu	• Healthy eyes • Cell growth • Potects against skin cancer • Boosts immune system • Essential for night vision	• Vitamins C, E • Zinc • Selenium • Multivitamin supplement	3,000 mcg 10,000 IU
1.2 mg	• Nerve growth • Converts food to energy, esp. fats • Memory • Cognition • Digestion	• All other B vitamins • Magnesium • Manganese	Not known
1.3 mg	• Makes red blood cells • Makes hormones • Releases energy from food • Helps regulate body acidity	• All other B vitamns • Selenium	Not known
16 mg	• Makes hormones • Removes toxins • Promotes normal cholestrol • Helps regulate blood sugar	• All other B vitamns • Chromium • Best taken with food	35 mg
5 mg	• Necessary to make vitamin D • Makes red blood cells • Makes hormones • Helps brain and nerve function	• All other B vitamns, esp. Biotin and Folc acid	Not known

VITAMIN	NAME	BEST PLANT SOURCES	BEST ANIMAL SOURCES	ADULT RDA/AI* WOMEN
B6 (water soluble)	Pyridoxine	• Peanuts • Beans • Peas • Bananas • Avocados • Potatoes • Whole grains	• Meat • Fish • Chicken • Milk	1.3 g
B7 (water soluble) (Vitamin H)	Biotin (Made by gut bacteria)	• Almonds • Oatmeal • Peanut butter • Bananas • Tomatoes • Corn • Grapefruit • Watermelon	• Liver • Egg yolks • Milk • Salmon • Oysters	30 mcg
B9 (water soluble)	Folic acid (folate)	• Dark green leafy veggies • Oranges • Beans • Avocados • Beets • Wheat germ	• Liver	400 mcg
B12 (water soluble)	Cobalamin	None	• Oysters • Chicken • Sardines • Tuna • Cottage cheese • Yogurt • Cheese • Eggs	2.4 mcg
Choline		Made by the body		400 mg

ADULT RDA/AI* MEN	IMPORTANT FOR:	VITAMINS AND MINERALS THAT HELP ABSORPTION	DAILY UPPER LIMIT
1.3 g	• Necessary for making proteins from amino acids • Makes enzymes • Prevents heart disease • Helps balance sex hormones • Helps nerves function • Promotes skin health	• All other B vitamins • Magnesium • Zinc	100 mg
30 mcg	• Breaks down food and converts to fuel • Essential during child development	• All other B vitamins • Magnesium • Manganese	Not known
400 mcg	• Necessary for cell growth and division • Prevents birth defects • Keeps arteries open • Promotes healthy moods • Promotes brain and nerve functions • Helps produce red blood cells	• All other B vitamins, esp. vitamin B12 • Vitamin C	1,000 mcg
2.4 mcg	• Processes protein into energy • Forms protective covering of nerve cells • Keeps red blood cells healthy • Prevents heart disease • Promotes healthy moods	• All other B vitamins • Calcium	Not known
550 mg	• Makes cell membranes • Helps liver metabolize fats	• Sold as PC-55 • In lecithin granules made from soybean oil • Similar to DMAE	3,500 mg

VITAMIN	NAME	BEST PLANT SOURCES	BEST ANIMAL SOURCES	ADULT RDA/AI* WOMEN
Inosital		• Citrus fruits • Nuts • Beans • Whole grains • Made by the body	• Organ meats	1,000 mg
PABA		• Wheat germ • Brown rice • Whole grains • Made by the body	• Liver	Not determined
C (water soluble)	Ascorbic acid	• Citrus fruits • Kiwi fruit • Strawberries • Melons • Cranberries • Papaya • Yellow peppers • Broccoli • Potatoes • Tomatoes	None	75 mg
D (fat soluble)	Calciferol	• Almost none • Sunlight	• Tuna, salmon sardines • Eggs • Cottage cheese • Milk	5–10 mcg 200–400 IU
E (fat soluble)	Tocopherol	• Almonds • Hazelnuts • Sunflower seeds • Wheat germ • Safflower oil	• Shrimp • Tuna	15 mg 22–100 IU
K (fat soluble) made by intestinal bacteria	Phylloqui-none	• Cauliflower • Dark green leafy veggies (kale, turnip and collard greens, broccoli)	• Beef liver • Eggs • Milk • Meat	90 mcg (1 mcg per kilo-gram of body weight)

ADULT RDA/AI* MEN	IMPORTANT FOR:	VITAMINS AND MINERALS THAT HELP ABSORPTION	DAILY UPPER LIMIT
1,000 mg	• Helps make neuro-transmitters • Helps diabetic neuropathy • May help depression, panic attacks		50 g
Not determined	• Blocks ultraviolet rays of the sun		1 g
90 mg	• Antioxidant • Needed to make collagen, which holds tissues together • Protects against cancer, heart disease, cataracts • Boosts immune system • Helps make antistress hormones • Helps heal wounds	• B vitamins • Vitamin E • Calcium • Magnesium • Bioflavinoids • Magnesium	2,000 mg – 4,000 mg (Note: RDA and upper limits of Vitamin C are subject of disagreement, esp. to combat illness)
5-10 mcg 200-400 IU	• Promotes bone & tooth health • Boosts immune system esp. T cells • Protects against colon cancer	• Dietary fat • Sunlight • Vitamins A, C, E protect D	50 mcg 2,000 IU
15 mg 22–100 IU	• Helps heart & vascular health • Helps prevent cancer • Boosts immune system • Protects against free radicals	• Dietary fat • Selenium • Vitamin A • Beta carotene • Vitamin C	1,000 mg almost 1,500 IU Note: if synthetic, 2,200 IU
120 mcg	• Promotes bone health • Makes blood clot		Not known

Note: Fat soluble vitamins are stored in the liver and fatty tissues, so you don't need to eat them every single day, and it is possible to take too much. Water soluble vitamins are not stored, so you have to eat them every day, and even better, spread intake over several meals of the day; it is unlikely for anyone to get too much.

*See "Essentials for Children," and "Essentials for Older Adults" and consult specialized nutrition books for RDA's for infants, children, and pregnant women. RDA=Recommended Daily Allowance; AI-Adequate Intake

** The liver converts beta carotenes into Vitamin A as needed.

6 Minerals

How Much We Need & Where To Get Them

MINERAL	BEST PLANT SOURCES	BEST ANIMAL SOURCES	ADULT RDA*
Calcium	• Green leafy veggies • Almonds • Parsley • Artichokes • Prunes	• Milk products • Ricotta cheese • Cheddar cheese • Swiss cheese	1,000 mg
Phosphorus (so widespread in food it is almost impossible to be deficient)	• Whole grains • Beans • Most vegetables • Nuts	• Meat • Eggs • Milk • Fish	1,000 mg
Magnesium	• Nuts (esp. brazil, almonds, cashews) • Beans • Dark green leafy veggies • Whole grains • Tofu • Chocolate	• Seafood • Milk • Beef liver • Eggs	300–420 mg
Zinc	• Beans • Nuts • Whole grains • Maple syrup (Note: plant-based zinc is poorly absorbed)	• Oysters • Shrimp • Lean meat • Organ meats • Turkey • Chicken	8 mg Men = 11 mg
Sodium Potassium Chloride (electrolytes) Sodium & Chloride are so common in all foods that deficiency is almost impossible	Sodium widely available, esp. table salt POTASSIUM: • Tomato juice • Beans • Avocado • Potatoes • Bananas • Cantaloupe • Orange juice • Molasses	POTASSIUM: • Meat • Milk • Cottage cheese	SODIUM: 1,300 mg POTASSIUM: 4,700 mg CHLORIDE: 2 g

IMPORTANT FOR:	VITAMINS & MINERALS THAT HELP ABSORPTION	DAILY UPPER LIMIT
• Promotes healthy bones & teeth • Helps blood clot • Prevents hypertension • Reduces PMS • Helps muscle contraction	• VitaminD • Vitamin K • Magnesium • Phosphorus • Boron	2,500 mg
• Promotes healthy bones & teeth • Builds muscle tissue • Helps balance body ph • Helps metabolism	• Calcium • Lactose • Vitamin D	Not determined
• Improves heart health; regulates heartbeats • Helps nerves to function • Manufactures enzymes • Causes muscle relaxation • Promotes healthy bones and teeth • Regulates body temperature • Promotes macronutrient metabolism	• Calcium • Potassium • Thiamin (B1) • Pyridoxine (B6) • Vitamin C • Vitamin D • Zinc • Phosphorus	350 mg from supplements
• Helps make enzymes and hormones and protein • Boosts immune system • Promotes wound healing • Helps fight colds • Promotes healthy skin, nails, and hair	• Vitamin A, B6, E • Magnesium • Calcium • Phosphorus	40 mg
• Keeps fluids in and between cells in balance • Carries nerve impulses • Helps muscles contract and relax • Moves nutrients into cells and waste out of cells • Regulates blood pressure and heartbeat	• Magnesium • Vitamin D	Not determined

MINERAL	BEST PLANT SOURCES	BEST ANIMAL SOURCES	ADULT RDA*
Boron	• Apples • Raisins • Pears • Grapes, dates	None	3–5 mg
Chromium	• Apples • Broccoli • Vegetable oils • Nuts • Mushrooms	• Beef • Egg yolks • Oysters	50–200 mcg
Cobalt	None known	• Meat • Eggs • Fish • Milk, yogurt • Cheese	2–4 mcg
Copper	• Nuts and seeds • Avocados • Potatoes • Whole grains • Beans • Prunes • Tomato juice	• Oysters • Lobsters • Beef liver	1.5–3 mg

Fluoride	• Added to water
	  and tooth paste
	• Tea
	• Plants from high
	  fluoride soils
		• Seafood	1.5–4 mg

Iodine	• Added to table salt	• Ocean fish • Milk	150 mcg
Iron	• Dark green vegetables • Whole grains • Peas and beans • Spinach • Nuts • Molasses	• Lean beef • Chicken • Oysters • Pork • Beef liver • Egg yolks	10–15 mg
Manganese	• Nuts • Tea • Raisins • Pineapple • Spinach • Lima beans • Whole grains • Beans • Leafy greens	None	1.8 mg Men = 2.3 mg

IMPORTANT FOR:	VITAMINS & MINERALS THAT HELP ABSORPTION	DAILY UPPER LIMIT
• Good for healthy bones – helps absorb calcium	Not known	Not determined
• Controls blood sugar • Helps builds muscle	Not known	Not determined
• Needed to make cobalamin (vitamin B12)	Not known	Not determined
• Helps circulation and artery health • Helps build nerve insulation • Necessary for antioxidant enzymes and red blood cells	Competes with zinc for absorption, should have 10 parts zinc to copper	10,000 mg
• Protects against tooth decay • Builds healthy bones		10 mg
• Needed for thyroid hormones		1,100 mg
• Needed for hemoglobin in red blood cells; helps blood carry oxygen	• Folic acid (B9) • Vitamin C, E • Phosphorus	45 mg
• Needed for protein digestion • Promotes connective tissue formation • Promates glucose absorption • Promotes healthy bones	• Zinc • Vitamins E, B1, C, K • Often in calcium supplements • High doses can interfere with iron absorption	11 mg

MINERAL	BEST PLANT SOURCES	BEST ANIMAL SOURCES	ADULT RDA*
Molybdenum	• Whole grains • Dark green veggies • Beans	• Lean meat • Milk	45 mcg
Nickel	• Chocolate • Whole grains • Nuts • Beans • Most fruits & vegetables	None	Not known
Selenium	• Brazil nuts • Whole grains • Oatmeal • Molasses	• Seafood • Lean meat • Chicken	55–70 mcg
Silicon	• Whole grains • Root vegetables • Beans	• Seafood	Not known
Sulfur	• Bean sprouts • Leafy greens • Raspberries • Beans and peas • Nuts	• Dairy products • Red meat • Egg yolks	Not known
Tin	Not known	Not known	Not known
Vanadium	Not known	Not known	Not known
Water	• Drinking water • Water in plant foods • Byproduct of metabolism	• Water in lean meat and fish	64 ounces daily

IMPORTANT FOR:	VITAMINS & MINERALS THAT HELP ABSORPTION	DAILY UPPER LIMIT
• Promotes normal growth and development • Helps make enzymes • Helps use iron • Removes toxins	• Dietary sulfur	2,000 mcg
• Needed to make certain hormones and enzymes • Protects healthy cell membranes	Not known	Not determined
• Needed for use of antioxidants, enzymes, glutathione • Reduces inflammation • Stimulates immune system	• Vitamins A, C, E	400 mcg
• Builds healthy bones, cartilage, connective tissue		Not determined
• Used in manufacture of amino acids and connective tissue • Helps regulate blood sugar levels	• Aids in manufacture of thiamin (Vitamin B1 and biotin [Vitamin B7])	Not determined
Unknown		Not known
Unknown		Not known
• Water is 2/3 of our body weight • Necessary for metabolism • Transport of nutrients • Maintain body temperature • Lubricant		

Trace Minerals – The minerals are needed in very tiny amounts and occur in a wide variety of foods. Also, most multivitamin and mineral supplements contain the recommended RDA for them.
* See "Essentials for Children," "Essentials for Older Adults," and consult specialized nutrition books for RDA's for infants, children, and pregnant women.
The following minerals are present in our bodies in small amounts, but there is no known need for them, and too much of them is harmful.
    Aluminum—In antacids
    Arsenic
    Cadmium
    Lead
    Mercury-found commonly in fish
*Check specialized lists for needs of special populations; e.g. pregnant or nursing women, older adults. Men need somewhat more zinc, magnesium, and manganese than women.

7 Superfoods

- Superfoods—foods that are so good for us, so full of healthy nutrients and so lacking in unhealthy properties—that they are superstars of a healthy diet.
- Most superfoods are plants--not surprising, because plants have the highest nutritional bang for the buck.

Most every nutrition writer has his or her favorite superfoods. I combined the superfoods lists of several writers and came up with 100 or so foods that would be good to eat several times a week. Hard to do.

So, I decided to list my 30 favorite Superfoods and divide them into the categories that make them so special: 1) rich in essential nutrients, 2) abundant vitamins and minerals, and/or 3) especially good at warding off heart disease and cancer.

My Top 30 Superfoods

A. Foods that are rich in **essential nutrients our bodies can't make:**

Beans and lentils	essential amino acids, complex carbs, fiber
Lean beef (grass fed)	rich in essential amino acids, and both saturated and unsaturated fats
Eggs (organic)	high amounts of essential amino acids and omega 3 fatty acids
Flaxseed (ground)	good source of omega 3 fatty acids
Walnuts	high in omega 3 fatty acids
High-fat wild fish (tuna, salmon, sardines, mackerel)	have abundant essential amino acids and omega 3 fatty acids

B. Foods that have especially high amounts of **many, many vitamins, minerals, and fiber:**

Greens (collards, turnip, dandelion)
Kale
Milk (organic)
Almonds
Olive oil (extra virgin)
Broccoli
Cabbage/Brussels sprouts
Oranges
Spinach
Sweet Potatoes
Whole grains, esp. wheat, barley, brown rice, quinoa

C. Foods that have **abundant antioxidants and anti-carcinogens;** these are heart-healthy; they lower cholesterol, support eye health, and boost immunity.

Apples
Blueberries
Cranberries
Strawberries
Garlic
Lemons
Oatmeal
Onions
Pomegranates
Tea (black and green)
Tomatoes
Wine (red)
Yogurt (with bioactive cultures)

Superfoods are easy to add to your diet:

1. Vegetables and fruit – eat as much as you want of unprocessed fruits and veggies {fresh or frozen). Mix up colors.
2. Grains – eat as much as you want of unprocessed grains (cooked). Limit processed grains like bread, pasta, and pastries.
3. Beans – eat as much as you want of cooked or frozen beans, peas, and lentils. (Canned are okay except those with lots of sugar.)
4. Dairy – eat low-fat milk products (not non-fat because with-

out fat the milk sugar lactose gets into your blood stream very quickly)-two servings a day.

5. Meat and poultry – add to diet sparingly; grass-fed beef and organic chicken are best.

6. Eggs – an egg a day is okay, or 6 a week.

Superfoods provide **dietary essentials:**
1. Essential amino acids
2. Essential fatty acids (including omega 3s)
3. Vitamins
4. Minerals
5. Fiber

Superfoods assist in **maintaining health:**

Digestion	Immunity boosters	Body integrity & functioning (skin, cell membranes, platelets, collagen, etc)	Vision
• Enzymes	• Antibacterial	• Essential fatty acids	• Cataracts
• Fiber	• Antiviral	• Protein	• Macular degeneration
	• Antifungal	• Hormones	
	• Anti-microbial		
	• Anti-toxins (pesticides)		

Superfoods help **prevent illness:**

Anti-Cancer	Anti-Heart Disease	Anti-Pain
• Antioxidants	• Antioxidants	• Anti-inflammatory
• Lignans	• Ant-hypertension	• COX-II inhibitors
• Sulfur	• Anti-obesity	
	• Lower LDL Cholesterol	
	• Anti-inflammatory	

8 Getting Protein From Plants

Omnivores—people who eat both animal and plant foods, usually don't have to worry about getting enough protein. In fact, many of us get far more than we actually need.

But vegetarians do want to make sure they are getting enough protein and, as it turns out, plants are a great source. Eating a varied plant diet virtually assures getting adequate protein.

Grains, nuts, and legumes (beans and peas) are all excellent sources of non-animal protein.

Recent research has found that it is not necessary to combine beans and grains in one meal to get complete protein. Eating both beans and grains over a day or two is adequate.

Top 20 Sources of Plant Protein
per ½ cup serving (unless otherwise noted)

GRAMS OF PROTEIN PER SERVING		CALORIES PER SERVING	
Tempeh (fermented tofu)	15.7	Tempeh (fermented tofu)	165
Soybeans (mature)	14.3	Soybeans (mature)	149
Edamame (young soybeans)	11.1	Edamame	127
Artichokes (1 med)	10.4	Artichokes (1 med)	150
Lentils	8.8	Lentils	115
Tofu, raw, firm	8.8	Tofu, raw, firm	91
Adzuki beans	8.6	Adzuki beans	147
Peanuts (1 oz.)	8	Peanuts (1 oz.)	170
Navy beans	7.9	Navy beans	129
Black beans	7.7	Black beans	114

GRAMS OF PROTEIN PER SERVING	CALORIES PER SERVING
Peanut butter (2 Tb) 7.7	Peanut butter (2 Tb) 188
Kidney beans 7.6	Kidney beans 113
Egg noodles 7.6	Egg noodles (enriched) 160
Spaghetti (ww) 7.5	Spaghetti (whole wheat) 174
Garbanzo beans 7.3	Garbanzo beans 135
Great N. beans 7.3	Great N. beans 105
Lima beans 7.3	Lima beans 108
Pinto beans 7	Pinto beans 117
Walnuts 6.9	Walnuts 172
Pine nuts 6.8	Pine nuts 160
Miso soup 5.3	Miso soup 140

As you can see, the top 20 sources of protein (above left) are not always the best choice if you are watching your calories. Some of the foods with the highest protein also are fairly high in calories.

If you want to maximize your protein intake for the least amount of calories, check out the table below. It is clear that green beans have the most protein per calorie; and, if you don't care for soybean products, legumes (beans, peas, lentils) are the best choice. The biggest surprise is artichokes, with more than 10 grams of protein per medium artichoke. But, go easy on the butter!

Top Twenty Sources of Plant Protein, relative to grams of protein per calorie

SERVING = 1/2 CUP (unless otherwise stated)	CALORIES	PROTEIN (g)	PROTEIN GRAMS PER CALORIE
Green beans	22	4.9	0.22
Tofu, raw, firm	92	9	0.10

SERVING = 1/2 CUP (unless otherwise stated)	CALORIES	PROTEIN (g)	PROTEIN GRAMS PER CALORIE
Soybeans (mature)	149	14.3	0.10
Tempeh	165	15.7	0.10
Edamame (immature soybeans)	127	11.1	0.09
Soymilk (8 ounces)	79	6.6	0.08
Lentils	115	8.8	0.08
Great Northern beans	105	7.3	0.07
Artichokes (1 med. cooked)	150	10.4	0.07
Broad beans	94	6.5	0.07
Lima beans	108	7.3	0.07
Black beans	114	7.7	0.07
Kidney beans	113	7.6	0.07
Peas	62	4.1	0.07
Wheat germ	104	6.7	0.06
Navy beans	129	7.9	0.06
Pinto beans	117	7	0.06
Adzuki beans	147	8.6	0.06
Tomatoes, sun dried (1/4 cup)	70	3.8	0.05
Garbanzo beans (chickpeas)	135	7.3	0.05

Regardless of which plants you choose to eat, there is no need to worry about getting enough protein if you choose to limit the amount of meat in your diet.Below are nutrient profiles for all the plant sources of proteins..

LEGUMES (BEANS, PEAS) (1/2 cup cooked)	CALORIES	PROTEIN (g)	FAT (g)	CARBS (g)	FIBER (g)
Adzuki beans	147	8.6	0.1	28	5.6
Black beans	114	7.7	0.5	20.4	7.5
Black-eyed peas	80	2.6	.04	15.7	4.2
Broad beans	94	6.5	0.05	16.7	4.6
Garbanzo beans (chickpeas)	135	7.3	2.1	23	6.3
Garbanzo beans (1/4 cup hummus)	210	6.1	10.4	25	6.3
Great Northern beans	105	7.3	.4	18.6	6.2
Kidney beans	113	7.6	0.5	20.2	6.5
Lentils	115	8.8	0.4	20	7.8
Lima beans	108	7.3	0.1	19.6	6.6
Navy beans	129	7.9	.05	24	5.8
Pinto beans	117	7	0.5	22	7.3
Peas	62	4.1	0.2	11.4	4.4
Green beans	22	4.9	0.2	4.9	2
Peanuts (1 ounce)	170	8	15	4	3
Peanut butter (2 Tbsp)	188	7.7	16	6.9	2.1

SOYBEAN PRODUCTS

(1/2 cup cooked)	CALORIES	PROTEIN (g)	FAT (g)	CARBS (g)	FIBER (g)
Edamame (immature soybeans)	127	11.1	5.8	9.9	3.8
Soybeans	149	14.3	7.7	8.5	5.2
Soymilk (8 ounces)	79	6.6	4.6	4.3	3.1
Tempeh	165	15.7	6.4	14.1	--
Tofu, raw, firm	91	8.8	11	5.4	2.9
Miso (4 fluid ounces)	284	16.3	8.4	38.6	7.5

NUTS & SEEDS
HIGH IN PROTEIN

(3 Tbsp)	CALORIES	PROTEIN (g)	FAT (g)	CARBS (g)	FIBER (g)
Almonds	166	5.6	14.6	5.7	3.1
Cashews	163	4.3	13.1	9.3	0.9
Flaxseed (1/4 cup)	93	3.3	6.3	7	1.6
Pine nuts	160	6.8	14.4	4	1.3
Pistachio nuts	172	4.2	15	7.8	3.1
Pumpkin seeds (1/2 cup)	110	5	5	14	2
Sesame seeds	161	4.8	13.6	7.4	4.8
Sunflower seeds	165	5.5	14.1	6.8	3.1
Walnuts	172	6.9	16	3.4	1.4

GRAINS, CEREALS, AND PASTA HIGH IN PROTEIN

	CALORIES	PROTEIN (g)	FAT (g)	CARBS (g)	FIBER (g)
Buckwheat groats (1/2 cup cooked)	91	3.3	6	20	2.8
Millet (1/2 cup cooked)	143	4.2	1.2	28.4	1.6
Quinoa (1/4 cup cooked)	159	5.5	2.5	29.3	2.5
Wild rice (1/2 cup cooked)	83	3.3	3	17.5	1.5
Wheat germ (1/4 cup cooked)	104	6.7	2.8	15	3.8
All Bran (1/2 cup)	81	3.9	1.1	23	10
Corn grits (1/4 cup dry)	140	3	5	31	1
Cream of Wheat (3 Tbsp dry)	120	3	0	25	1
Oatmeal (1/2 cup dry)	148	5.5	3	27.3	3.7
Raisin Bran (1/2 cup)	97	3	7	23.5	4.1
Egg noodles (enriched) (1 cup cooked)	160	7.6	2.4	39.7	1.8

GRAINS, CEREALS, AND PASTA HIGH IN PROTEIN	CALORIES	PROTEIN (g)	FAT (g)	CARBS (g)	FIBER (g)
Spaghetti (enriched) (1 cup cooked)	197	6.7	9	39.7	2.4
Spaghetti (whole wheat) (1 cup cooked)	174	7.5	8	37.2	6.3

VEGETABLES FAIRLY HIGH IN PROTEIN	CALORIES	PROTEIN (g)	FAT (g)	CARBS (g)	FIBER (g)
Artichokes (1 medium cooked)	150	10.4	0.5	33.5	16.2
Avocado (1 medium)	306	3.7	30	12	8.5
Potato (1 medium baked)	212	4.9	0.2	48.7	4.6
Tomato (sun dried) (1/4 cup)	70	3.8	0.8	15	3.3

Sources: Hark, Lisa and Darwin, Deen. *Nutrition for Life*. DK. 2005; Neoporent, Liz and Schlosberg, Suzanne. *The Fat-Free Truth*. Houghton-Mifflin. 2005;

9 Phytochemicals
So That's Why Plants Are So Good For Us

- Plants are full of chemical compounds called phytochemicals or phytonutrients (phyto is from the Greek, pertaining to plants). There are literally thousands of these substances, most of which science knows little about.
- Phytochemicals are not essential nutrients and are not required by the body to sustain life. But some are known to support the body's normal functioning, as well as performing a protective function, defending us from diseases caused by damage to our cells—from toxins in food and air, to free radicals left over from digesting food.
- Whole grains, dark green leafy vegetables, cruciferous vegetables (cabbage, broccoli, cauliflower), soybeans, onions and garlic, tomatoes, fruits, tea, wine, and some herbs and spices are thought to contain particularly beneficial amounts of phytochemicals.
- Some of the well-known phytochemicals are lycopene in tomatoes, isoflavones in soy and beta carotenes in yellow and orange vegetables.

What phytochemicals do:
- **Antioxidants and anti-cancer** – Allyl sulfides (onions, leeks, garlic), carotenoids (fruits, carrots), flavonoids (fruits, vegetables), polyphenols (tea, grapes).
- **Hormonal action** – Isoflavones, found in soy, imitate human estrogens and help to reduce menopausal symptoms and osteoporosis.
- **Stimulation of enzymes** – Indoles, which are found in cabbages, stimulate enzymes that make the estrogen less effective and could reduce the risk for breast cancer. Other phytochemicals, which interfere with enzymes, are protease inhibitors (soy and beans), and terpenes (citrus fruits and cherries).
- **Interference with DNA replication** – Saponins found in beans interfere with the replication of cell DNA, thereby preventing the

multiplication of cancer cells. Capsaicin, found in hot peppers, protects DNA from carcinogens.
- **Anti-bacterial effects** – The phytochemical allicin from garlic has anti-bacterial properties.
- **Cellular action** – Some phytochemicals bind physically to cell walls, thereby preventing the adhesion of pathogens to human cell walls. Proanthocyanidins are responsible for the anti-adhesion properties of cranberries. Consumption of cranberries reduces the risk of urinary tract infections and may improve dental health.

The four main classes of phytochemicals are:
1. **Phenols** – A group of more than 4,000 plant pigments that give many plants their intense colors. They seem to have a protective effect against heart disease and stroke, as well as anti-bacterial and anti-carcinogenic effects.
2. **Organo-sulfides** – Compounds that provide a boost to the immune system by anti-bacterial and anti-carcinogenic actions, particularly colon, breast, and digestive system cancers. The most famous is allium in garlic.
3. **Terpenes** – Carotenoids, phytosterols, and saponins. Well known carotenoids are lycopene and lutein, and, of course, beta carotene, all of which provide protection against vascular eye disease, and many forms of cancer. Phytosterols function like estrogens, providing protection against breast, prostate, and ovarian cancers, and heart disease. Lignans are a form of phytosterol.
4. **Indoles** – Abundant in cruciferous vegetables (broccoli, cabbage, cauliflower, Brussels sprouts, kale), indoles confer powerful anti-carcinogenic effects. The allium in garlic is an indole.

Below is a *selected* list of common phytochemicals and the foods in which they are abundant. It is not known whether phytochemical supplements are effective in the same way as the phytonutrients you get directly from plants. In any case, these are compounds you are likely to find in your favorite health food store.

NAME	TYPE	POSSIBLE BENEFITS	BEST FOOD SOURCES
Anthocyanidins/ Proanthocyanidids	Bioflavinoid	• Fights gout and arthritis	Berries, grapes, currants
Boswellic acid	Anti-inflammatory	• Arthritis	Frankincense
Capsaicin	Anti-inflammatory	• Protects against DNA damage • Helps arthritis pain	Hot chili peppers
Carotenoids	Antioxidant	• Neutralizes free radicals and protects against heart disease	Yellow & orange fruits & veggies Carrots Sweet potatoes Oranges Peas
Chlorophyll		• Stimulates blood cell production in bone marrow • Protects again radiation • Kills germs • Wound healer	Wheat grass Algae Seaweed Green leafy veggies
Courmarins Chlorogenic acid		• Prevents formation of nitrosamines, which are carcinogenic	Tomatoes Green peppers Pineapple Strawberries Carrots
Curcumin	Polyphenol	• Binds to free radicals • Protects against cancer and heart disease	Mustard Turmeric Corn Yellow peppers Ginger
Ellagic acid	Polyphenol	• Neutralizes carcinogens • Prevents formation of nitrosamines in meat and aflatoxin in peanuts	Strawberries Raspberries Blueberries Walnuts Pomegranates Garlic
Genistein Daidzein	Isoflavones	• Inhibits growth of breast, ovarian, colon, and prostate cancers • Strengthens bones • Fights menopause symptoms	Soy milk Tofu Legumes (beans, peas)

NAME	TYPE	POSSIBLE BENEFITS	BEST FOOD SOURCES
Glucosinolates	Indole	• Protection for many cancers • Helps liver detoxify • Protection from heart disease	Broccolini Broccoli Brussels sprouts Cabbage Cauliflower
Hesperidin, Rutin	Bioflavinoids	• Binds to toxic chemicals • Stablizes vitamin C in tissues • Antibiotic • Anti-carcinogenic • Helps bleeding gums, varicose veins, hemorrhoids, bruises	Citrus fruit Berries Broccoli Cherries Grapes Papayas Cantaloupe Tea Red wine Tomatoes
Isothiocyanates (ITCs) and other Indoles	Indoles	• Powerful cancer protector, esp. estrogen-promoted cancers • Kills cancer cells • Inhibits growth of cancer cells	Broccolini Broccoli Brussels sprouts Cabbage Cauliflower Kale Kohlrabi Mustard Radishes Turnips
Lentinan	Anti-carcinogen	• Induces production of the antiviral interferon	Shiitake mushrooms
Lignans	Phytosterol	• Binds to estrogen receptors to fight breast, colon, ovarian, and prostate cancers	Flaxseeds Sunflower seeds Beans Nuts
Limoene	Monoterpene	• Protects lung tissue from damage	Citrus peels Cherries
Lutein	Carotenoid	• Helps prevent age-related macular degeneration (AMD)	Green leafy veggies Cabbage Spinach Kale Broccoli Cauliflower

NAME	TYPE	POSSIBLE BENEFITS	BEST FOOD SOURCES
Lycopene	Carotenoid	• Anti-cancer properties esp. esophageal, stomach, and prostate cancers • Preserves eyesight	Tomatoes Watermelon Red peppers
Organosulfides	Sulfide	• Stimulates anticancer enzymes and slows the formation of blood clots, boosts immune system	Onions & leeks
Sterols Stanols	Phytosterols	• Lowers LDL cholesterol by inhibiting absorption of cholesterol	Seeds Beans Lentils Seed oils
Piperine		• Facilitates uptake of nutrients from food	Black pepper Chilis Paprika Cayenne
Quercetin	Bioflavinoid	• Lowers symptoms of hay fever, eczema, asthma • Inhibits release of histamines • Anti-inflammatory • Anti-bacterial • Anti-carcinogenic • Protects capillaries • Protects connective tissue	All berries, esp. strawberries Tea Buckwheat Citrus fruit
Resveratrol	Bioflavinoid	• Anti-carcinogenic • Anti-inflammatory • Fights cardiovascular disease	Red grapes Red wine
Sulphoraphane	Isothiocyanate	• Anti-bacterial • Prevents stomach ulcers	Broccoli Cauliflower Brussel sprouts Kale Ginger Onions
Zeanxanthin	Cartenoid	• Neutralizes free radicals to fight cardiovascular disease • Protects eye health	Corn Spinach Cabbage Broccoli Peas Grapes Kale Turnip greens Egg yolks

The following outline shows the relationship of selected phytochemicals to each other. Use it as a handy reference guide for supplements you find at your favorite health food store.

Phenolic compounds

Monophenols – parsley, rosemary, oregano, thyme, dill

Polyphenols (Bioflavonoids) – red, blue, purple pigments

- **Flavonols**
  - Anthocyanins and Anthocyanidins – red wine, red, purple or blue fruits and vegetables
  - Quercetin – red and yellow onions, tea, wine, apples, cranberries, beans
  - Kaempferol – strawberries, cranberries, peas, cruciferous vegetables, chives
  - Myricetin – grapes, walnuts
  - Rutin – citrus fruits, buckwheat, parsley, tomato, apricot, rhubarb, tea
- **Flavanones**
  - Hesperidin – citrus fruits
  - Naringenin – citrus fruits
- **Flavan-3-ols**
  - Catechins – white, green, and black tea, grapes, wine, cocoa, lentils, black-eyed peas
  - Cyanidin – red apple & pear, blackberry, blueberry, cherry, cranberry, peach, plum
  - Phytoestrogens
  - Daidzein (formononetin) – soy, alfalfa sprouts, chickpeas, peanuts, other legumes
  - Genistein (biochanin A) – soy, alfalfa sprouts
  - chickpeas, peanuts, other legumes
  - Glycitein – soy
  - Coumestrol – red clover, alfalfa sprouts, soy, peas, brussels sprouts

Phenolic acids

- **Ellagic acid** – walnuts, strawberries, cranberries, blackberries, guava, grapes
- **Gallic acid** – tea, mango, strawberries, rhubarb, soy

- **Salicylic acid** – peppermint, licorice, peanut, wheat
- **Tannic acid** – nettles, tea, berries
- **Vanillin** – vanilla beans, cloves
- **Capsaicin** – chili peppers
- **Curcumin** – turmeric, mustard (Oxidizes to vanillin)

Lignans (phytoestrogens) – seeds (flax, sesame, pumpkin, sunflower, poppy), whole grains (rye, oats, barley), bran (wheat, oat, rye), fruits (particularly berries) and vegetables

- **Silymarin** – artichokes, milk thistle
- **Matairesinol** – flax seed, sesame seed, rye bran and meal, oat bran, poppy seed, strawberries, blackcurrants, broccoli
- **Secoisolariciresinol** – flax seeds, sunflower seeds, sesame seeds, pumpkin, strawberries, blueberries, cranberries, zucchini, black-currant, carrots

Tyrosol esters

- **Tyrosol** – olive oil
- **Oleocanthal** – olive oil
- **Oleoropein** – olive oil

Stilbenoids

- **Resveratrol** – grape skins and seeds, wine, nuts, peanuts
- **Pterostilbene** – grapes, blueberries
- **Piceatannol** – grapes

Terpenes (isoprenoids)

Carotenoids (tetraterpenoids)

- **Carotenes - orange pigments**
  - alpha(α)-Carotene – to vitamin A, in carrots, pumpkins, maize, tangerine, orange
  - Beta(β)-Carotene – to vitamin A, in dark, leafy greens and red, orange and yellow fruits and vegetables
  - Phytofluene – star fruit, sweet potato, orange
- **Xanthophylls - yellow pigments.**
  - Canthaxanthin – paprika
  - Cryptoxanthin – mango, tangerine, orange, papaya, peaches, avocado, pea, grapefruit, kiwi
  - Zeaxanthin –spinach, kale, turnip greens, eggs, red pepper, pumpkin, oranges

- Astaxanthin – microalge, yeast, krill, shrimp, salmon, lobsters, and some crabs
- Lutein – spinach, turnip greens, romaine lettuce, eggs, red pepper, pumpkin, mango, papaya, oranges, kiwi, peaches, squash, legumes, broccoli, cauliflower, cabbage, prunes, sweet potatoes, honeydew melon, rhubarb, plum, avocado, pear

Saponins – soybeans, beans, other legumes, maize, alfalfa

Lipids

- **Phytosterols** – almonds, cashews, peanuts, sesame seeds, sunflower seeds, whole wheat, maize, soybeans, many vegetable oils
- **beta Sitosterol** – avocados, rice bran, wheat germ, corn oils, fennel, peanuts, soybeans, hawthorn, basil, buckwheat
- **Tocopherols** (vitamin E)
- **omega-3, 6,9 fatty acids** – dark-green leafy vegetables, grains, legumes, nuts

Organosulfides

Dithiolthiones (isothiocyanates)
- **Sulphoraphane** – broccoli, cauliflower, cabbage
- **Thiosulphonates** (allium compounds)
- **Allyl methyl trisulfide** – garlic, onions, leeks, chives, shallots
- **Diallyl sulfide** – garlic, onions, leeks, chives, shallots

Indoles, glucosinolates

Indole-3-carbinol – cabbage, kale, Brussels sprouts, rutabaga, mustard greens

Sulforaphane – broccoli family

Sinigrin – broccoli family

Allicin – garlic

Allyl isothiocyanate – horseradish, mustard, wasabi

Piperine – black pepper

Adapted from "phytochemicals" from the Linus Pauling Institute of Oregon State University (lpi.oregonstate.edu) and Wood, Frank K. Eat and Heal. FC&A Medical Publishing. 2004.

10 All About Fats

Like carbohydrate and protein, dietary fat is essential for life. Here's what the fat in our bodies does for us:

- Fat is fuel—the body metabolizes dietary and stored body fat for energy, just like carbs and proteins
- Dietary fat facilitates the absorption of fat-soluble vitamins
- Essential fatty acids are necessary for tissue formation, child growth and development. Our bodies can't make these fats, so we have to eat them
- Body fat insulates our bodies and provides cushioning
- Body fat lubricates body tissues and slows loss of water from tissues and pores
- Fat, in the form of cholesterol, helps digestion since it is a component of bile salts
- Fat, as cholesterol, helps build healthy cell membranes, especially important for brain functions
- Fat, as cholesterol, is necessary in the production of hormones (cortisone, adrenalin, estrogen, testosterone)

Clearly, without fat we could not sustain life. But, most of us eat much more fat than our bodies need, largely because

- fat makes food taste good—it is the primary enhancer of flavor:
- many processed foods contain a very high proportion of fat, and we eat a lot of highly processed and prepared foods
- fat is digested more slowly than carbohydrates and proteins, so fat helps us avoid hunger between meals

Three types of dietary fat

The fat in foods is classified as;

1. Saturated – from animals and seed oils and vegetable oils
2. Monounsaturated – mostly from olive and sesame oils
3. Polyunsaturated – mostly from plants and vegetable oils

How Much?

There is little agreement on the optimal proportion of fats in the diet relative to proteins and carbohydrates. For our purposes, let's assume a good balance for most healthy people is 40% carbs, 30% protein, and 30% fat.

Your total fat intake should be divided in thirds among three types of fat. If your total fat allowance for the day is 65 grams, then your saturated fat intake should be less than 16 grams, your polyunsaturated fat intake less than 23 grams, and your monounsaturated fat intake between 20 and 26 grams.

Recommended Fat Intake by Percent (based on 65 grams per day)

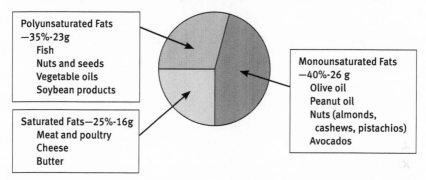

Polyunsaturated Fats
—35%-23g
  Fish
  Nuts and seeds
  Vegetable oils
  Soybean products

Monounsaturated Fats
—40%-26 g
  Olive oil
  Peanut oil
  Nuts (almonds,
    cashews, pistachios)
  Avocados

Saturated Fats—25%-16g
  Meat and poultry
  Cheese
  Butter

Saturated and monounsaturated fats are not essential in our diets—the body can manufacture them. They perform critical functions in the body and are a source of energy. Polyunsaturated fats are essential. The body can't manufacture them; we must get them from the food we eat.

Plant and animal sources of fat usually contain all three types of fat, but in vastly varying proportions. For example:

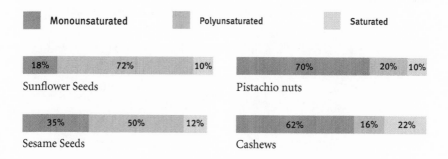

Monounsaturated   Polyunsaturated   Saturated

| 18% | 72% | 10% |
Sunflower Seeds

| 70% | 20% | 10% |
Pistachio nuts

| 35% | 50% | 12% |
Sesame Seeds

| 62% | 16% | 22% |
Cashews

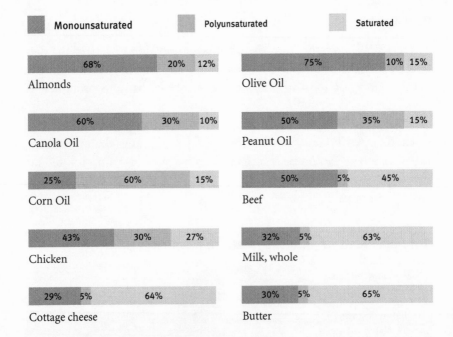

Monounsaturated   Polyunsaturated   Saturated

68%   20%   12%
Almonds

75%   10% 15%
Olive Oil

60%   30%   10%
Canola Oil

50%   35%   15%
Peanut Oil

25%   60%   15%
Corn Oil

50%   5%   45%
Beef

43%   30%   27%
Chicken

32%   5%   63%
Milk, whole

29%   5%   64%
Cottage cheese

30%   5%   65%
Butter

Polyunsaturated fats come in two forms:

1. **OMEGA 3** – Alpha-linolenic acid (ALA)– found in flax, hemp and pumpkin seeds, and walnuts

    Omega 3's are converted into EPA – (eicosapentaenoic acid) also found in oily fish

    EPA is converted into DHA (docosahexaenoic acid) also found in oily fish

    - EPA and DHA are both precursors of PGE_3 (non-inflammatory prostagladins), which *help* the body to function.

2. **OMEGA 6** – Linoleic acid – found in sunflower, sesame, safflower seeds and corn;

    Omega 6's are converted into GLA (gamma-linolenic acid) also found in walnuts, soybeans and wheat germ, and in borage and evening primrose oils, used in supplements

    GLA is converted into AA (arachidonic acid) also found in meat and milk

    - GLA is the precursor to PGE_1 (non-inflammatory prostagladins) – also *helpful* to bodily functions.
    - AA is the precursor to PGE_2 (inflammatory prostaglandins), which are *harmful*, causing inflammation and pain.

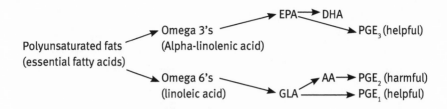

If you shop for supplemental forms of EPA, DHA, and GLA, these confusing abbreviations are what you usually find. Now you know what they mean and where they come from.

A healthy balance of omega-3 and omega-6 fatty acids is essential because they both make prostaglandins, hormone-like substances needed to regulate many body processes. The ratio of omega 3 to omega 6 in our diet should be between 1:1 and 1:4. Most people get about 1:20, because of high omega 6's in processed foods

- PGE_1 prostaglandins regulate blood pressure, heart rhythms, kidneys, and digestion.
- PGE_3 are essential for proper brain function, control cholesterol, maintain fluid balance, and reduce stickiness of blood;
- Acute inflammation and swelling are normal consequences of injury to tissues. However, chronic inflammation causes ongoing injury to tissues and results from an excess of inflammatory prostaglandins (PGE_2). A diet that is out of balance with respect to polyunsaturated fats is one cause of chronic inflammation.

Good Food Sources of Omega 3's and Omega 6's

ALA – ALPHA-LINOLENIC ACID (FROM OMEGA 3 FATTY ACIDS)	EPA AND DHA (FROM ALA)	GLA (FROM OMEGA 6-LINOLEIC ACID) most people get more than enough
• Flaxseeds & flaxseed oil	• Albacore tuna	• Flaxseeds
• Soybeans & soybean oil	• Sardines	• Corn & corn oil
• Walnuts	• Salmon	• Sunflower seeds & oil
• Brazil nuts	• Mackerel	• Sesame seeds & oil
• Soy nuts	• Atlantic herring	• Walnuts
• Olive oil	• Swordfish	
• Hemp seeds	• Lake trout	
• Pumpkin seeds		

There are many other types of fatty acids—oleic acid, palmitic acid, butyric acid, lauric acid which are nonessential because your body can manufacture them. They are found in olive and peanut oils, in avocados, coconuts, and nuts. In small quantities, all provide healthy benefits.

Trans fatty acids

Trans fatty acids are rare in nature. They are created only in the rumen of cows and sheep, and are found only in small amounts in milk, cheese, beef and lamb. One, called Conjugated Linoleic Acid (CLA), has been studied extensively and seems to confer protection from elevated cholesterol in the blood, lowers insulin resistance to prevent diabetes, inhibits production of inflammatory prostaglandins, and has antioxidant properties.

Most dietary trans fatty acids come from manufactured foods (margarine and similar spreads), and produce unhealthy effects in humans: elevated LDL cholesterol, inflammation, sticky platelets. Extra hydrogen atoms are injected into mono and polyunsaturated fats, causing them to behave like saturated fats in the body, facilitating the production of plaque in arteries. Look for products that have less than one per cent trans fatty acids on the label.

Sources: Holford. *Optimum Nutrition*, and Enig, *Eat Fats, Lose Fat;* Hark. *Nutrition for Life.* Willett, Walter C. *Eat, Drink, and Be Healthy.* Free Press. 2001.

11 Antioxidant Superstars

- Many vitamins, phytochemicals, and other nutrients function as antioxidants, protecting our cells from damage caused by free radicals.
- Free radicals occur as a natural result of digestion and metabolism but can also come from environmental toxins such as smoking, pesticides, pollution and radiation.
- Antioxidants neutralize free radicals, so they become inactive and no longer a threat to our health.
- See "Phytochemicals" (Chapter 9) for more information about antioxidants.

	ANTIOXIDANTS ORAC* UNITS PER SERVING
Blueberries — 1/2 cup	1620
Blackberries — 1/2 cup	1466
Prunes — 3 prunes	1386
Broccolini — 1/2 cup cooked	1159
Kale — 1/2 cup cooked	1150
Strawberries — 1/2 cup	1144
Spinach — 1/2 cup cooked	1089
Raisins — 1/4 cup	1019
Orange — 1 medium	982
Broccoli — 1/2 cup cooked	817
Raspberries — 1/2 cup	755
Beets — 1/2 cup cooked	715
Spinach — 1/2 cup raw	678
Cantalope — 1/2 small melon	670
Baked beans — 1/2 cup cooked	640

*ORAC Measurements:

1. Antioxidants are measured in ORAC Units – oxygen radical absorbance capacity.
2. ORAC Units were developed by the Nutrition Center at Tufts University in Boston.

3. The daily requirement for antioxidants is 3,500 ORAC units; 5,000 to 6,000 units will provide optimal protection against cancer, heart disease, and aging. Five servings of fruits and vegetables should meet this requirement easily.

More Foods High in Antioxidants

FOOD	ONE SERVING	ANTIOXIDANTS IN ONE SERVING
Grapefruit, pink	1/2 grapefruit	580
Red pepper	1 medum pepper	540
Kiwi fruit	1 kiwi	458
Cherries	10 cherries	455
Beans, kidney	1/2 cup cooked	400
Onion	1/2 cup chopped	360
Corn	1/2 cup cooked	330
Apple, Red Delicious	1 medium apple	300

Sources: Holford, Patrick. The New Optimum Nutrition Bible. The Crossing Press. 2004; and Bowden, Jonny. 150 Healthiest Foods on Earth. Fair Winds Press, 2007.

12 Fiber In Your Food

Fiber is all those parts of plants that our bodies can't digest—mostly cell walls, skins, and seed coverings. But that doesn't make those parts useless to us.

Fiber. . .

- absorbs water from food
- facilitates the transit of stool through the colon and bowel, allowing less time for toxins (pesticides, bile acids, food additives and preservatives, heavy metals, chemical pollutants) to be absorbed, as well as preventing bowel problems
- slows the transit of nutrients through the small intestine, stabilizing the rate of glucose metabolism
- prevents some cholesterol from being absorbed by the small intestine

Two types of fiber in plants:

1. **Insoluble (35%)** – the cellulose of cell walls, seed covers (bran), and rough stems of celery and broccoli are all insoluble. They absorb water, but don't dissolve in it. Water-saturated cellulose helps keep stool soft so it can move easily through the colon and bowel, preventing problems like constipation, diverticulitis, colon cancer, and hemorrhoids.
2. **Soluble (45%)** – the skins and rinds of fruits and vegetables contain in their cells a substance called pectin, and some seeds, beans, grains, and nuts contain mucilage, called guar gum, also used as a thickener in processed foods. Pectin and mucilage dissolve in water to form a gel in your intestines This gel can trap toxins and some of your body's natural cholesterol in your small intestine, preventing absorption. The gel also can slow the transit and absorption of carbohydrates to prevent blood sugar spikes after eating.

How much? Nutrition experts believe that we should get 11.5 g of fiber for every 1,000 calories we eat, or about 25–30 g per day at a minimum. The average American eats about 12 g of fiber per day.

Good Sources of Fiber

INSOLUBLE FIBER	SOLUBLE FIBER
Artichokes	Apples
Broccoli	Carrots
Carrots	Cauliflower
Dried beans and peas (cooked)	Citrus fruits
Nuts	Corn
Parsnips	Dried beans
Popcorn	Lentils
Potatoes (with skin)	Oat bran
Seeds (sunflower, sesame, flax)	Oatmeal
Sweet potatoes (with skin)	Pears
Wheat bran	Rice bran (in brown rice)
Whole grains	Sweet potatoes

Note: Fiber supplements can increase your daily fiber without adding calories. Take supplements in the early evening for most predictable benefits. Just in case fiber interferes with vitamin and mineral absorption, take multivitamins at a different time than fiber supplements.

Some easy ways to increase your daily fiber intake:

1. Sprinkle wheat germ and/or flax seeds on your morning cereal.
2. Add a dash of seeds—sunflower, sesame, pine nuts—to salads and rice dishes.
3. Add a serving or two of legumes (beans, peas, lentils) to your routine menu plans.
4. An apple a day. . . .
5. Make oats a routine part of breakfast several times a week.
6. Eat sweet potatoes with skin as often as white potatoes.

13 Probiotics

A lot of talk about probiotics stems from widespread ads on TV for yogurt products for which health claims are made for improving digestion and "regularity."

Here's what the **National Institutes of Health** has to say: (www.nih.gov)

1. Probiotics are living microorganisms (in most cases, bacteria) that are similar to beneficial microorganisms found in the human gut. (Microorganisms are tiny living organisms—such as bacteria, viruses, and yeasts—that can be seen only under a microscope.)
2. Most often, the bacteria come from two groups, *Lactobacillus* or *Bifidobacterium*, including their subspecies *lactobacillus acidopholus* and *bifidobacterium bidifus*. A few common probiotics, such as *Saccharomyces boulardii*, are yeasts, which are different from bacteria.
3. Some probiotic foods date back to ancient times: fermented foods like miso, sauerkraut and pickles and cultured milk products (yogurt and kefir).
4. Probiotics are not the same thing as prebiotics [which are] non-digestible food ingredients that stimulate the growth of beneficial microorganisms already in people's colons.
5. Probiotics are available to consumers mainly in foods (soy products, fermented milk products) and dietary supplements. Interest in probiotics in general has been growing; Americans' spending on probiotic supplements, for example, nearly tripled from 1994 to 2003.

Normally, bodies are populated by hundreds of microorganisms—in and on the skin, in the gut, and in other orifices. Friendly bacteria are vital to proper development of the immune system, to protection against disease-causing bacteria, and to the digestion and absorption of food and nutrients. Each person's particular mix of bacteria varies. An individual's normal bacterial balance can be thrown off by:

1. Taking antibiotics, which can kill friendly bacteria in the gut, along with unfriendly bacteria. Some people use probiotics to try to offset side effects from antibiotics like gas, cramping, or diarrhea.
2. "Unfriendly" microorganisms can invade the body, such as bacteria, yeasts, fungi, and parasites, which can cause
    - Infectious diarrhea and irritable bowel syndrome
    - Inflammatory bowel disease (e.g., ulcerative colitis and Crohn's disease)
    - Infection with Helicobacter pylori (H. pylori), a bacterium that causes most ulcers and many types of chronic stomach inflammation
    - Tooth decay and periodontal disease
    - Vaginal infections
    - Stomach, skin, and respiratory infections that children acquire in daycare

According to NIH
1. There is limited evidence supporting some uses of probiotics. Much more scientific knowledge is needed about probiotics, including about their safety and appropriate use.
2. Effects found from one species or strain of probiotics do not necessarily hold true for others, or even for different preparations of the same species or strain.

14 Sweeteners
Natural and Artificial

Why we love sweets
1. Humans are hard-wired to love sweets: we are born with a preference for foods that taste sweet.
2. Some scientists believe this is because naturally-occurring sweet foods are generally highly nutritious, or they contain lots of calories needed for energy.
3. Nutrition and energy were both necessary in the diets of primitive humans.

Where do natural sweets come from?
1. There is some form of sugar in many plants, particularly root vegetables (glucose) and fruits (fructose).
2. When these plants are highly refined into what we know as table sugar (sucrose), the nutrients are stripped away, leaving just the calories.
3. To avoid the "empty calories" of sucrose, many people seek out less refined sugar substitutes (see below) Minimal refining leaves some nutrients, especially minerals, and fiber, which makes them less harmful than sugar, because they are metabolized more slowly.
4. Unrefined sweeteners often have greater sweetness than table sugar, meaning fewer calories per serving.
5. Milk is another source of natural sugar (lactose).

NATURAL SWEETENERS

Agave Nectar	From the sap of the agave plant; light grade has neutral flavor; darker grades have strong, earthy flavor; one and a half times sweeter than sugar; similar to honey, but does not involve insect pollination. Same calories as sugar, but you need less.

Barley Malt Syrup	Made from sprouted barley; contains maltose and glucose, dark brown, similar to molasses. Half as sweet as white sugar. Good with sweet root vegetables and used for malted drinks.
Blackstrap Molasses	Dark syrup left over from the table sugar refining process; contains the vitamins and minerals sugar refining leaves behind, esp. calcium, iron, potassium. Strong flavor but not as sweet as sugar; comes in light and dark strengths.
Brown Rice Syrup	Made from brown rice; heavy amber syrup like butterscotch; half as sweet as sugar; contains maltose and complex carbs and most nutrients of brown rice. Use like honey.
Date Sugar	From ground dried dates; mostly dark brown coarse moist grains; use in combination with sugar for baking. Sucrose and fructose. High in folic acid. Can't be used in liquids as the grains don't dissolve.
Evap. White Grape Juice	White grape juice evaporated into whitish grains; must be kept in airtight container or it turns stone-hard.
Fructose	From fruits; resembles granular white sugar but is more concentrated; less is needed—about 1/2 cup fructose to 1 cup of sugar. Has little nutritional value; use like table sugar.
Fruit Juice Concentrate	Made from apples, cranberries, peaches, pears, grapes, and pineapple; some natural fructose; mostly sucrose; fruity flavor; use in baking.
Honey	Made from flower nectar by bees; contains fructose, glucose, and sucrose; flavors and sweetness vary by plant source; can be half again as sweet as sugar.
Maple Sugar	Dehydrated granules of maple syrup. Mostly sucrose; use like sugar.
Maple syrup	Boiled down from sap of maple trees; 60% sucrose; light to dark brown with distinctive maple flavor; high in potassium and calcium. About 2/3 as sweet as sugar.
Stevia	From the stevia shrub; 300 times sweeter than sugar; widely available; Comes in powder and liquid; Zero calories; slight aftertaste.
Sucanat	The name is a contraction of suger-cane-natural, and it's basically unrefined sugar or dehydrated sugar cane juice, but with no remaining nutrients; similar to brown sugar; mild molasses flavor
Sucrose (table sugar)	Highly refined, mostly from sugar cane and sugar beets.

Acesulfame-K (Sunette and Sweet One)	200 times sweeter than table sugar; zero calories; can be used for baking; has a bitter taste on its own.
Aspartame (Equal & NutraSweet)	180 to 200 times sweeter than table sugar; one gram of aspartame contains 4 calories; cannot be used for baking
Saccharin (Sweet'N Low)	300 times sweeter than table sugar; made from petroleum; zero calories; can be used for baking; comes in individual packets and liquid form.
Sorbitol, Mannitol, Xylitol	Sugar alcohols that occur naturally in fruits; commercially made for use as sweeteners; absorbed slowly. Some parts aren't absorbed at all, so consuming these in large quantities may cause diarrhea.
Sucralose (Splenda)	600 times sweeter than table sugar; zero calories; can be used for baking; contains maltodextrin to bulk it up; comes in individual packets, bulk granules, and blended with brown sugar.

Names often found in ingredients lists which all mean sugar:

Brown sugar	Invert sugar
Corn sweetener	Lactose
Corn syrup	Maltose
Dextrose	Malt syrup
Fructose	Molasses
Fruit juice concentrates	Raw sugar
Glucose	Sucrose
High-fructose corn syrup	Sugar
Honey Syrup	Turbinado

Sources: www.livrite.com/sweeten
www.grist.com
www.care2.com/greenliving/directory-of-natural-sweeteners.html
www.usda.gov

15 Go for the Grains

NUTRITION SUPERSTARS	WHY
Whole wheat	The most popular and versatile grain of all. In its unprocessed form, it has abundant protein, vitamins, minerals, and fiber. Every part of the grain can be used. Its flour has been made into literally hundreds of different products. Unfortunately, in its most popular form—highly refined white flour—it has been stripped of most of its nutrients and besides calories, has little nutritive value.
Quinoa	Highest protein and calcium of any grain except whole wheat; high in fiber and exceptionally rich in choline, potassium, and folate
Oatmeal	Excellent source of cholesterol lowering soluble fiber; rich in folate, and exceptional in lutein supporting eye health
Brown rice	Good source of protein and low in carbs; rich in choline and magnesium for heart health

LOWEST CALORE GRAINS (IN ORDER)	
Sweet Corn	70 per ½ large ear
Brown Rice	70 per ½ cup cooked
Oatmeal	71 per ½ cup cooked
Buckwheat	78 per ½ cup cooked
Wild Rice	82 per ½ cup cooked

HIGHEST FIBER GRAINS (IN ORDER)	
Whole wheat	3.6 g per ½ cup cooked
Quinoa	3 g per ½ cup cooked
Barley	3 g per ½ cup cooked
Buckwheat groats	2.7 g per ½ cup cooked

Degrees of Grain Processing

Grains are milled either minimally, which removes just the outer covering, or maximally, which results in fine flour. Some grains are best eaten whole or minimally processed; others lend themselves to being rolled into flakes for cereals, or ground fine for baking, as meal or flour. Below is a description of processing styles, from least to most.

Generally, the least amount of processing results in the most nutritious grain product, highest in vitamins, minerals, and fiber, and lowest in calories per serving.

Whole Grains
- undergoes the least amount of processing; only the outer hull is removed
- require the longest cooking time
- are the most nutritious form of grain because the nutrient-rich bran and germ are left intact.
- are also referred to as hulled grains.
- example: whole wheat

Pearled
- refers to the removal of the bran layers resulting in grain with much less fiber
- cooks faster and is more tender than whole grain.
- also known as polished grain
- example: pearled barley

Grits
- a form of grain in which the whole kernels have been cut into smaller pieces
- they cook much more quickly
- grits are also known as steel-cut or cracked grains
- examples: hominy grits; steel-cut oats

Grain Flakes
- created with a process in which the grain is steamed and rolled to produce flattened, or flaked kernels, allowing the grain to cook at a much faster rate
- Grain flakes are also known as rolled grains
- examples: ready to eat flake cereals; rolled oats

Meal
- refers to grain that has been ground until it has a coarse, sandy texture
- often used in breads and cereals
- examples: cornmeal; Malt-O-Meal cereal

Flour
- a form of grain created by grinding and sifting grain into a powdered form
- varies from very soft to coarse in texture
- used as the main ingredient for making most baked goods: breads, cakes, pastries, etc.

- examples: all purpose flour, cake flour, rye flour

Certain parts of the whole grain are sold separately because they are highly nutritious.

Bran
- the nutrient-packed layers covering the inner kernel of grain.
- basically indigestible, but loaded with fiber
- Some types of bran are so popular as a food supplement that they are sold as a separate product
- Sometimes bran is removed during processing and ground into a meal to be used as a supplement or food additive
- examples: wheat, oat and rice bran

Germ
- the embryo of a kernel of grain, located at the bottom center of the kernel
- the oily part of a kernel or seed from which a new plant sprouts.
- loaded with vitamins and minerals so it is highly nutritious
- also contains fat, which decreases the shelf life of the grain and any grain product containing the germ
- example: wheat germ

Following are nutrient profiles for most grains popular in the western diet.

Wheat

Varieties of wheat are categorized by:

1. **Kernel Hardness:** Hard wheat varieties are high in protein. The more protein in the wheat, the more gluten is formed when flour milled from the wheat is combined with liquid. Gluten provides dough with elasticity and the ability to stretch as the leavening agent produces carbon dioxide gas, which enables dough to rise effectively. Soft wheat varieties have less protein than hard wheat, so the gluten forming capacity of the flour milled from soft wheat is not as great, making soft wheat flour a good choice for cakes and pastries.
2. **Bran Color:** The bran is the fibrous outer layers of the inner kernel that are either a variation of red or white.
3. **Growing Season:** Spring wheat is planted in the spring and har-

vested in the late summer and fall in locations where the winters are cold. Winter wheat is best suited to locations where the winters are shorter and less severe. It is planted during the autumn months, lies dormant during the winter, sprouts in the late winter or early spring, and is ready for harvesting in the early summer.

In the United States, the basic classifications of wheat are:

1. **Hard Wheat:** varieties of hard wheat include hard white, hard red winter, and hard red spring, all of which are used for yeast breads and similar products. The protein content of hard wheat usually ranges from 10 to 14 percent.
2. **Soft Wheat:** varieties of soft wheat include soft white and soft red winter, which are both used for products such as cakes, cookies, and pastries that do not require the same level of leavening capability as yeast breads. The protein content of soft wheat varieties usually ranges from 6 to 10 percent.
3. **Durum:** the hardest wheat grown. Durum wheat is used almost exclusively for making pasta and is most often ground into a granular flour with a light yellow color known as semolina, which has the ideal properties for making the best pasta. (Italian pasta makers never refer to semolina as flour - they refer to it as grain.) Durum is high in protein and gluten, which are necessary for making good pasta. It is occasionally used for baked goods (especially risen breads).

Hard Whole Wheat Nutrients per 1/2 cup

PROTEIN	CARBS	FAT	FIBER	HIGH IN THESE VITAMINS	HIGH IN THESE MINERALS	KCALS
8.2 g	44g	1 g	7.3 g	Niacin 3.8 mg Choline 18.5 ? Folate 27 mcg Vitamin K 1.2 mcg Beta Carotene 3 mg Lutien + Zeaxanthin 132 mcg	Calcium 20 mg Iron 2.3 mg Magnesium 83 mg Manganese 1.9 mg Phosphorus 207 mg Potassium 243 mg Sodium 3 mg Selenium 9 mcg Zinc 1.8 mg	203

Specialty Grains Related to Wheat

Kamut

- closely related to durum wheat and is often considered a specialty grain
- kernels are 2 to 3 times larger than a typical wheat kernel
- has a nutty, buttery flavor and is sold as a whole grain, as flour, and in the form of flakes
- excellent in soups, salads, pilafs, or savory side dishes
- also found in commercially prepared cereals, crackers, and breads and pastas

Spelt (Farro)

- American variety is called spelt; European is called farro
- similar in taste to barley
- the hull adheres to the grain when harvested, similar to barley and oats
- processed in whole or cracked form; the texture differs considerably when cooked
- used for polenta and bread recipes
- provides a nutty flavor to salads, soups, stews, side dishes, and meat stuffing

Take a look at the list below for some other grains worth a try as you vary your diet to include more whole grains:

Amaranth

- not actually a grain, but an herb used as a grain
- amaranth seed (or grain) is light tan in color and has a very mild tangy or peppery flavor.

Amaranth Nutrients per cup (flakes)

PROTEIN	CARBS	FAT	FIBER	HIGH IN THESE VITAMINS	HIGH IN THESE MINERALS	KCALS
6 g	27 g	2.7 g	4 g	Choline 29 mg Niacin 2 mg Folate 4 mcg Lutien + Zeaxanthin 86 mcg	Calcium 6 mg Magnesium 10 mg Phosphorus 126 mg Potassium 134 mg Selenium 27 mcg	134

Barley

- has a nutty and somewhat sweet flavor
- color ranges from a light tan to various shades of brown or purple
- hulled barley, also called barley groats, has only the outer covering of the grain removed
- hulled barley is commonly used for cereal
- pearl barley has the hull and bran removed so it cooks faster
- use pearled barely in soups and salads for texture contrasts

Barley Nutrients per 1/2 cup (cooked)

PROTEIN	CARBS	FAT	FIBER	HIGH IN THESE VITAMINS	HIGH IN THESE MINERALS	KCALS
1.8 g	23 g	.4 g	3 g	Vitamin A 7 IU Choline 11 mg Niacin 2 mg Folate 13 mcg Beta carotene 4 mg Lutien + Zeaxanthin 91 mcg	Calcium 9 mg Iron 1.7 mg Magnesium 18 mg Phosphorus 44 mg Potassium 75 mg Selenium 8 mcg	99

Brown Rice

- has a chewy texture and a nutty flavor
- use the same ways as white rice, as a side dish, in soups and paired with veggies

Brown Rice Nutrients per 1/2 cup (cooked)

PROTEIN	CARBS	FAT	FIBER	HIGH IN THESE VITAMINS	HIGH IN THESE MINERALS	KCALS
5 g	22 g	.8 g	2 g	Choline 9 mg Niacin 1.5 mg Folate 4 mcg	Calcium 10 mg Magnesium 42 mg Phosphorus 80 mg Potassium 42 mg Selenium 9 mcg Sodium 294 mg	114

Buckwheat

- Buckwheat groats have an earthy, grassy flavor with a slight cocoa taste and taste best when the kernels are roasted; roasted buckwheat is called "Kasha"
- A native plant of Russia, buckwheat is actually an herb that is related to rhubarb and sorrel
- Buckwheat seeds are used for hot cereal, sausage filler, soups, and savory side dishes
- Buckwheat is most often ground into flour and used in pancakes, crepes, muffins, and soba noodles

Buckwheat Nutrients per 1/2 cup (cooked)

PROTEIN	CARBS	FAT	FIBER	HIGH IN THESE VITAMINS	HIGH IN THESE MINERALS	KCALS
2.9 g	17 g	.5 g	2.7 g	Vitamin A 7 IU Choline 17 mg Folate 12 mcg Vitamin K 1.5 mcg Lutien + Zeaxanthin 50 mcg	Calcium 6 mg Magnesium 43 mg Phosphorus 59 mg Potassium 74 mg Selenium 2 mcg	78

Sweet Corn

- There are several varieties of corn (dent corn, flint corn, popcorn, flour corn) which vary by the amount of moisture in the kernels.; some are used for animal feed, others for specialized applications such as corn meal, tortillas, etc.
- Sweet corn is the variety commonly used as a vegetable in human diets. Sweet corn has a higher sugar content than other types of corn
- The three most common types of sweet corn are white corn (white kernels), yellow corn (yellow kernels), and a hybrid of both white and yellow, often referred to as peaches and cream or butter and sugar corn

Sweet Corn Nutrients per ear (large)

PROTEIN	CARBS	FAT	FIBER	HIGH IN THESE VITAMINS	HIGH IN THESE MINERALS	KCALS
4 g	29 g	3.5 g	3.2 g	Vitamin A 26 mcg Vitamin C 7.1 mg Niacin 2 mg Choline 34 mg Folate 52 mcg Vitamin K 4 mcg Lutien + Zeaxanthin 1032 mcg Beta carotene 96 mg	Calcium 5 mg Magnesium 30 mg Phosphorus 86 mg Potassium 243 mg Sodium 284 mg	140

Flax

- grown for its fiber and seeds
- not really considered a grain (like amaranth and buckwheat)
- The small, brown seeds are most often used as a food additive because of the delicious nutty flavor and the nutritional benefits

Flaxseed Nutrients per 2 tablespoons (18 g)

PROTEIN	CARBS	FAT	FIBER	HIGH IN THESE VITAMINS	HIGH IN THESE MINERALS	KCALS
4 g	6 g	8.1 g	6.8 g	Choline 34 mg Folate 52 mcg Lutien + Zeaxanthin 118 mcg	Calcium 46 mg Magnesium 70 mg Phosphorus 116 mg Potassium 146 mg Sodium 6 mg Selenium 5 mcg	96

Millet

- tiny seeds range in color from bright yellow to rust, depending on the variety
- was an important food staple in Europe and Asia, and still is in developing countries in Africa
- today in the United States, millet is most often used as a popular variety of birdseed

- has a mild sweetness and crunchy texture
- eaten as a cereal, a side dish, polenta, and as an addition to soups and stews and desserts
- seeds are especially good when toasted

Millet Nutrients per 1/2 cup (cooked)

PROTEIN	CARBS	FAT	FIBER	HIGH IN THESE VITAMINS	HIGH IN THESE MINERALS	KCALS
3 g	20 g	8 g	1 g	Niacin 1 mg Choline 10 mg Folate 16 mcg Lutien + Zeaxanthin 61 mcg	Calcium 3 mg Magnesium 36 mg Phosphorus 88 mg Potassium 54 mg Sodium 15 mg	103

Oats

- colors of the different varieties range from light beige or yellow grains to reddish-gray and black
- oat grains are processed to remove the outer hull, but the nutritious bran and germ are kept
- processing includes steaming, rolling, cutting, and grinding to produce products such as oat bran, oat flakes, oatmeal, steel cut oats, rolled oats, and oat flour

Oatmeal Nutrients per cup (cooked)

PROTEIN	CARBS	FAT	FIBER	HIGH IN THESE VITAMINS	HIGH IN THESE MINERALS	KCALS
5 g	26 g	2.5 g	4 g	Choline 15 mg Folate 9 mcg Lutien + Zeaxanthin 61 mcg	Calcium 26 mg Magnesium 54 mg Phosphorus 147 mg Potassium 131 mg Sodium 283 mg Selenium 11 mcg Zinc 1.4 mg	143

Quinoa

- not a true grain, but the seeds are used as one
- part of the same botanical family as beets
- the plant produces clusters that contain thousands of tiny bead-shaped seeds that range in color from light beige to yellow to rust to almost black
- cooked seeds increase in size 3 or 4 times, and become tender, with a springy texture

Quinoa Nutrients per 1/2 cup (cooked)

PROTEIN	CARBS	FAT	FIBER	HIGH IN THESE VITAMINS	HIGH IN THESE MINERALS	KCALS
6.5 g	35 g	3 g	3 g	Choline 15 mg Folate 25 mcg	Calcium 30 mg Iron 4.5 mg Magnesium 105 mg Phosphorus 205 mg Potassium 370 mg Sodium 10 mg Zinc 1.6 mg	180

White rice

- an important part of the diet of half the world's population—nearly 50% of daily calories
- grown in river deltas, flooded or irrigated coastal plains, or terraced hillsides
- the husk, bran, and germ have been removed (polished), which allows it to cook rapidly

White Rice Nutrients per cup (cooked)

PROTEIN	CARBS	FAT	FIBER	HIGH IN THESE VITAMINS	HIGH IN THESE MINERALS	KCALS
2 g	22 g	.2 g	.3 g	Choline 1.6 mg Folate 45 mcg Niacin 1.2 mg	Calcium 8 mg Magnesium 10 mg Phosphorus 34 mg Potassium 23 mg Sodium 284 mg Selenium 6 mcg	90

Rye

- has a very assertive and hearty flavor with a slightly bitter taste
- color of the grain may range from beige to dark gray
- processed into a variety of forms including whole kernels (berries), flakes, meal, and flour
- whole grains require longer cooking times than other grains. soaking the berries overnight decreases the cooking time
- rye berries are used in stews, rice, and vegetable stir-fries
- rye flour is available in varieties ranging from light to dark and textures ranging from course to fine
- used in the creation of various alcoholic beverages, such as whiskey, because it ferments quickly

Rye Nutrients per cup (cooked)

PROTEIN	CARBS	FAT	FIBER	HIGH IN THESE VITAMINS	HIGH IN THESE MINERALS	KCALS
2.5 g	24 g	.2 g	4.3 g	Choline 3.3 mg Folate 5 mcg Vitamin K 1.8 mcg Lutien + Zeaxanthin 55 mcg	Calcium 13 mg Magnesium 23 mg Phosphorus 55 mg Potassium 68 mg Sodium 351 mg Selenium 10.5 mcg	108

Sorghum

- a cereal plant native to Africa, but cultivated in many parts of the world
- sometimes confused with millet
- grain ranges in color from white to red; white grain is used as a food source; the red grain is used for livestock feed
- grain has a sweet, nutty flavor, delicious when steamed or added to soups and casseroles

Sorghum Nutrients per 1/2 cup (cooked)

PROTEIN	CARBS	FAT	FIBER	HIGH IN THESE VITAMINS	HIGH IN THESE MINERALS	KCALS
5.8 g	37 g	1.6 g	3 g	Not available	Calcium 14 mg Iron 2.2 mg Phosphorus 143 mg Potassium 68 mg Sodium 3 mg Selenium 10.5 mcg	170

Triticale

- a high protein man-made grain produced by crossbreeding wheat and rye
- duplicates the protein and bread-making merits of wheat and the durability and high lysine content of rye
- grain doesn't taste like rye, but it has a stronger, nuttier flavor than wheat
- excellent for breads and other baked goods

Triticale Bread Nutrients per slice

PROTEIN	CARBS	FAT	FIBER	HIGH IN THESE VITAMINS	HIGH IN THESE MINERALS	KCALS
2.7 g	11 g	.8 g	1.6 g	Choline 5.2 mg Folate 20 mcg Vitamin K 1.1 mcg Lutien + Zeaxanthin 16 mcg	Calcium 22 mg Magnesium 15 mg Phosphorus 41 mg Potassium 52 mg Sodium 142 mg Selenium 9mcg	63

Wild rice

- not actually a type of rice, but an aquatic grass bearing edible seeds that grows wild in marshy areas of lakes and rivers
- after harvesting, wild rice is dried and roasted, or parched, to loosen the hull, which is removed
- color may range from varying shades of yellow, tan, brown, to almost black, and is darkened by roasting

- wild rice has such a distinctive flavor that a small quantity is sufficient to provide adequate flavor to rice blends
- used as an ingredient for soups and casseroles. A small quantity added to steamed vegetables makes an excellent side dish. It adds flavor to tossed salads and goes well with poultry and fish

Wild Rice Nutrients per 1/2 cup (cooked)

PROTEIN	CARBS	FAT	FIBER	HIGH IN THESE VITAMINS	HIGH IN THESE MINERALS	KCALS
3.3 g	18 g	.3 g	1.5 g	Niacin 1.1 mg	Calcium 2.52 mg	82
				Choline 8.3 mg	Magnesium 26 mg	
				Folate 21 mcg	Phosphorus 68 mg	
				Beta carotene 3 mg	Potassium 82 mg	
				Lutien + Zeaxanthin	Sodium 290 mg	
				52 mcg	Zinc 1.2 mg	

16 Dark Green Leafy Vegetables

NUTRITION SUPERSTARS	
Kale	Highest of all vegetables in antioxidants; rich in cancer-fighting indoles and sulforaphane; high in bone-building calcium and vitamin K and offers a high amount of fiber.
Collard greens	Excellent source of lutein and zeaxanthin for eye health; exceptionally high in fiber (5 g per cup), beta carotene, vitamin C, calcium, and potassium.
Spinach	High in iron and vitamin K; excellent source of anti-cancer flavonoids; calcium is poorly absorbed because of high oxalic acid content of spinach.
Broccoli	Phytochemicals called isothiocyanates neutralize carcinogens in the body—brocolli and other members of the cruciferous family have the most isothiocyanates of all vegetables. Rich in indoles which stimulate detoxifying enzymes, and sulforaphane for prostate health.
Purslane	Unfamiiar to most Americans, purslane boasts the highest amount of omega 3 fatty acids of any green vegetable, and has exceptional amounts of vitamin A, calcium, and potassium. Grows as a weed throughout the U.S., but some farmers markets and specialty stores may carry it.
Dandelion leaves and roots	A weed to most of us, dandelions boast an exceptional nutrient storehouse, especially for stimulating chemicals that detoxify the liver and help the gall bladder release bile, an aid in digestion. Inulin in dandelion root increases insulin sensitivity in diabetics, and cholesterol lowering pectin. Cooked greens contain the highest amount of beta carotene and vitamin A of all green vegetables.

Dark green leafy greens are . . .

- Low in calories, super high in nutrients, dark green leafy vegetables are nutritional powerhouses, perhaps the most concentrated source of nutrition of any food.

- Leafy greens boast exceptional quantities of vitamins A, K, C, E, many of the B vitamins, particularly folate and minerals (especially iron, calcium, potassium, and magnesium).
- A variety of phytonutrients are found in leafy greens, including beta-carotene, lutein, and zeaxanthin, and cancer fighting indoles. Dark green leaves even contain small amounts of omega-3 fats and a surprising amount of fiber in their stems.
- Greens are very low carb, and the carbs are packed in layers of fiber, which make them very slow to digest. That is why greens typically have very little impact on blood glucose and are not counted in many diet plans.

IMPORTANT: always eat greens with a small amount of fat because many of the nutrients are fat soluble as in salad dressing, cooking oil or butter, cheese, and nuts.

Some Easy Ways to Add Greens to Your Diet

1. **Salads** – Small, tender leaves, both mild and pungent, add texture and flavor interest to your salads.
2. **Soups:** Try mixing collard or beet greens, kale or mustard greens into your favorite soups.
3. **Stir-fry:** Add chopped leafy greens or broccoli to your stir-fried meals, with or without meat.
4. **Steam** hearty leaves like collard greens, kale, or spinach. Add water to a pot and place a steamer with the vegetables into it. Bring the water to a simmer, cover with a lid, and wait a few minutes until your vegetables are slightly soft. Add a bit of butter or oil, salt and pepper for a great side dish.
5. **Sauté** chopped leaves in a frying pan with a small amount of good oil and some garlic if you like; takes only a minute or two, and reduces the volume a lot.
6. **Braise** hearty, large leaves in a small amount of liquid and your favorite seasonings; cover and simmer
7. **Casseroles:** Add blanched greens to casseroles and egg dishes before cooking.

Flavors That Go Well with Greens

- Smoked meats, including bacon, sausage, proscuitto, and smoked turkey
- Lemon, vinegar and Worcestershire Sauce
- Hot chiles in any form (dried pepper flakes, hot sauce, etc.)
- Anchovies
- Cream and/or cheese

SALAD/SANDWICH GREENS	
Arugula	Radicchio
Cabbage	Purslane
Dandelion	Sorrel
Endive	Spinach
Escarole	Spring greens
Iceberg lettuce	Watercress
Romaine	

COOKING GREENS	
QUICK COOKING	SLOWER COOKING
Spinach	Broccoli
Swiss chard	Kale
Cabbage	Collard greens
Beet greens	Beet greens
Bok choy	Mustard greens
	Turnip greens
	Kohlrabi greens

Easy Salad Dressing

It's easy to make your own dressing right in the salad bowl. Start with vinegar (any kind is good, but balsamic is really good), lemon juice or lime juice — add salt, pepper and seasonings as desired (garlic and herbs). Let this soak for as much time as you have. Whisk in some oil (two or three times as much oil as vinegar) just before assembling the salad ingredients. Alternatively, you can do the same thing in a small jar.

Tip: While assembling salad greens, throw a handful of mixed, chopped nuts in a fry pan on medium heat, shake occasionally while making the salad, add to salad before dressing.

Now that you know how, try adding some of these greens to your menu for new taste and texture adventures:

Artichoke

- hearts and bases of leaves have a mild, buttery flavor (even without dipping in butter)

- aids in digestion by provoking production of bile
- among the highest protein of all plants (10 g per medium artichoke)
- detoxifies liver
- rich in magnesium, potassium, lutein, and fiber

Arugula

- has a pungent, peppery taste
- is rich in vitamins A, C, K and calcium
- can be eaten raw in salads or added to stir-fry, soups, and pasta sauces

Bok Choy

- has a sweet, mild grassy flavor
- is rich in potassium, calcium, beta carotene, vitamin A and fiber
- great in soups, or sautéed in a mixture of spinach and chard
- rich in cancer fighting indoles and isothiocyanates

Broccoli

- has both soft florets and crunchy stalks, with a slightly bitter flavor
- is rich in vitamins A, C, and K, folate, potassium, calcium, lutein, and fiber
- rich in cancer fighting indoles and isothiocyanates
- can be eaten raw, steamed, sautéed or added to a casserole
- Peeled stalks taste sweet and mild, very different than florets, and make great crudite, or chopped in salads

Broccoli Rabe

- distantly related to broccoli, closer to turnips
- peppery, aggressively bitter flavor; blanching tames the flavor
- add to pasta, soups, casseroles to spice them up
- rich in cancer fighting indoles, sulforaphane, and bioflavonoids and fiber
- nutrition powerhouse: calcium, potassium, vitamins A, C, and K, folate, lutien and zeaxanthin

Brussels Sprouts

- taste a bit like cabbage, but sweeter
- high in isothiocyanates and sulforaphane, anti-cancer agents
- rich in vitamins A, C, and K, folate, potassium, calcium, lutein
- best steamed and sprinkled with nutmeg

Cabbage (red and green)

- king of the cruciferous veggies for anti-cancer properties
- extremely versatile - eaten both raw in slaws, and cooked with other veggies and meats
- indoles increase the ration of "good" estrogen metabolites to "bad" estrogen metabolites
- red variety contains anthocyanins, which are powerful anti-inflammatory antioxidants
- rich in calcium, magnesium, potassium, vitamins C and K, beta carotene, and lutein

Collard Greens

- have a mild flavor; take well to high-flavored seasonings
- are rich in vitamins A, C and K, folate, fiber, and calcium
- boil them briefly and then add to a soup or stir-fry, or combine with beans
- also eat collard greens as a side dish. Just sauté with your favorite seasonings

Dandelion Greens

- have a bitter, tangy flavor
- exceedingly rich in vitamin A, beta carotene and calcium
- used widely to detoxify the liver and stimulate bile production
- best when steamed or eaten raw in salad
- contain inulin and pectin, soluble fibers that increase calcium and magnesium absorption
- is a natural potassium-sparing diuretic which might help lower blood pressure

Endive/Escarole

- fresh and slightly bitter taste
- small, sturdy but tender leaves and a mild taste make these leafy greens excellent in salads
- not a nutrient superstar, but high in folate, and good amounts of vitamins A and K, beta carotene, calcium, iron, potassium

Kale

- has a slightly bitter, cabbage-like flavor
- is rich in vitamins A, C and K, calcium, iron, beta carotene, and lutein and zeaxanthin
- highest of all vegetables in antioxidants and cancer-fighting indoles and sulforaphane
- tasty when added to soups, stir-fries, and sauces, or combined with starchy veggies

Kohlrabi greens

- leaves taste similar to cabbage
- contain all the cancer-fighting compounds—indoles, sulforaphane, and isothiocyanates
- rich in vitamin C and potassium
- Blanch leaves and add to soups, or braise with turnip, mustard or collard greens and your favorite seasonings.

Mustard Greens

- have a peppery or spicy flavor
- are rich in vitamins A, C, and K, folate, and calcium
- delicious when eaten raw in salads or in stir-fries and soups.

Purslane

- leaves have a mild, sweet and sour flavor and chewy texture
- grows wild all over the United States, but many consider it a weed

- exceptionally nutritious source of antioxidants and omega-3 fatty acids
- rich in calcium, potassium, and vitamin A
- use raw in salads, or steamed and added to soups, stews, and other steamed veggies

Romaine

- a nutrient rich lettuce that is high in vitamins A, C, and K, calcium, and folate
- best when eaten raw in salads, sandwiches or wraps

Spinach

- has a sweet flavor
- a nutritional powerhouse, rich in vitamins A, C and K, manganese, folate, magnesium, beta carotene, and iron
- contains quercetin, a powerful antioxidant and anti-inflammatory
- tastes great eaten raw in salads, or steamed, or sauteed

Swiss Chard

- comes in red and white varieties
- tastes similar to spinach
- is rich in vitamins A, C, and K, potassium and iron
- exceptionally high in vitamin A and beta carotene, and lutein and zeaxanthin.
- delicate leaves are best quickly sautéed or stir-fried or eaten raw in salads

Turnip Greens

- related to cabbage, with the same cancer-fighting indoles and iso-thiocyanates
- greens are exceptionally high in vitamins A and K, calcium, beta carotene, and lutein and zeaxanthin

- blanch and add to soups, stews, or steamed root veggies, or braise with other hearty greens and your favorite seasonings

Watercress

- has a more pungent, stimulating flavor than you'd expect from these tender leaves
- has four times the calcium and six times the magnesium of milk, as much vitamin C as oranges, and more iron than spinach
- particularly rich in vitamins A and K, beta carotene, and lutein
- a member of the cruciferous vegetable family, it has the same cancer-fighting nutrients indoles and isothiocyanates

17 Nuts and Seeds

NUTRITION SUPERSTARS	
NUTS	
Walnuts	only nut that contains significant amount of omega 3 fatty acids
Pistachio nuts	best nut source of beta carotene; high potassium-to-sodium ratio for heart health
Almonds	more calcium than any other nut; high in protein and fiber
Macadamia nuts	most amount of monounsaturated fat than any other nut
SEEDS	
Flax seeds	best plant source of omega 3 fatty acid; high in protein & fiber
Sunflower seeds	high in vitamin E and selenium
Pumpkin seeds	rich in cholesterol-lowering phytosterols
Sesame seeds	contain high amounts of lignans that enhance vitamin E absorption

PRIMARY NUTRIENTS IN MOST NUTS & SEEDS		HEALTH BENEFITS OF NUTS
Unsaturated fats	Calcium	Decrease serum (blood) cholesterol
Fiber	Magnesium	Reduce hypertension
Vitamin E	Phosphorus	Decrease inflammation
Polyphenols	Potassium	Delay or prevent onset of Type II diabetes

NUTS

Almonds

- The almond fruit is the edible seed of sweet almond trees.
- High in monounsaturated fat (70%). Almonds have more calcium than any other nut and are an excellent source of iron, riboflavin, and vitamin E. There are 6 g of protein and 3 g of fiber in an ounce.

- Almonds come whole, sliced, flaked, and slivered. Almond oil, extracted from the kernel of the Bitter Almond, is used for flavoring and for skin care preparations. Almond milk is a highly nutritious dairy milk substitute.

Beechnuts

- Beechnuts are enclosed in prickly burrs that fall from beech trees in the autumn. They look like small chestnuts and taste like hazelnuts.
- Beechnuts are an excellent source of thiamin and riboflavin and a good source of iron. Monounsaturated and polyunsaturated fats provide more than 80% of the fat content.

Brazil Nuts

- Brazil nuts, also known as the para nut, butternut, cream nut, and castanea, grow only in South America.
- 12-24 nuts grow inside a hard, woody fruit similar to a coconut shell.
- Brazil nuts are rich, creamy, and sweet and are one of the richest sources of dietary selenium, a potent anti-carcinogenic.

Cashews

- Cashews are higher in protein and carbohydrate than many nuts.•
- They are not sold in the shell because the shells are covered by caustic oil which can burn the skin.
- Nutritionally, cashews are an excellent source of phosphorus and a good source of potassium.
- The primary source of fat in cashews is monounsaturated fat.

Chestnuts

- Chestnuts are used in soups, fritters, porridges, stuffings and stews, as well as being roasted or boiled whole.
- Available fresh in autumn, they are also dried, canned — whole or pureed, or ground into flour.

- High in starch, but low in protein and fat, chestnuts are rich in folate and minerals, especially potassium..

Coconuts

- The coconut palm is common in tropical regions all over the world.
- Every part of the fruit is edible and nutritious. Unripe nuts contain coconut milk. Nutmeat can be eaten fresh or dried. Oil is extracted from the nut meat and used for cooking and margarines.
- Coconut fats are almost entirely saturated, but of a different, healthier type than the saturated fats from animals.

Ginkgo Nuts

- The ginkgo nut is the seed of an inedible, apricot-like fruit that is well known for its strong, some might say offensive, odor.
- Nuts borne from female trees are soft with a delicate, sweet taste.
- Although the ginkgo tree is common in the U.S., many people are unaware that it bears edible nuts.
- Extracts and powders derived from ginkgo leaves are popular herbal supplements, promoted as a memory aid.
- Ginkgo nuts are low in fat and protein and an excellent source of vitamin A, phosphorus, potassium, copper, thiamin, and niacin.

Hazelnuts (Filberts)

- Hazelnuts are an excellent source of calcium and magnesium and contain a plant sterol beta-sitosterol, shown to lessen symptoms of benign prostatic hyperplasia.
- Monounsaturated fat is the predominant source of fat in hazelnuts.

Lotus Seeds

- The roots, seeds, and leaves of the lotus plant are edible. Lotus seeds, also known as hasu and nelumbium, have a delicate, mild flavor.

- Lotus seeds are lower in calories and higher in carbohydrates than most other seeds. Rich in potassium, their fats are mostly polyunsaturated.

Macadamia Nuts

- Macadamia nuts' slightly sweet, creamy, rich flavor and crunchy texture have acquired a "gourmet" reputation.
- The fat in the macadamia nut is 80% heart healthy monounsaturated fat, higher even than olive oil.
- Macadamia nuts are an excellent source of magnesium, calcium, and thiamin and a good source of iron and niacin.
- These nuts also contain phytosterols, including beta-sitosterol, which helps lower cholesterol and the symptoms of benign prostatic hyperplasia.

Peanuts

- Peanuts are not actually nuts, but legumes.
- Peanuts are high in protein, a rich source of potassium, and are fairly high in folate. Peanut butter shares the same nutritional profile, as long as it does not contain added hydrogenated oils.
- Peanuts are very high in antioxidants and fiber, both heart healthy and possibly anti-carcinogenic.

Pecans

- Pecans are elongated and wrinkled, resembling a walnut, and have a rich, sweet, buttery flavor.
- Most of the fat in pecans is monounsaturated.
- Pecans are an excellent source of phosphorus, thiamin, copper, and zinc and a good source of calcium, iron and potassium.

Pistachio Nuts

- Pistachios' hard, thin, tan shell partially splits open when the nut is ripe.
- The nut is a smooth, pale-green kernel wrapped in a fine brown-

ish skin, with a delicate and sweet flavor, which lends itself to desserts.
- Pistachios are an excellent source of vitamins A and E, beta carotene, iron, magnesium, phosphorus, potassium, and thiamin. The main source of fat in pistachios is monounsaturated fat.
- Rich in phytosterols, especially beta-sitosterol, which can lower cholesterol and support prostate health.
- Pistachios have a very high potassium to sodium ratio, which helps normalize blood pressure and maintain water balance. And vitamin E boosts the immune system.

Walnuts

- Walnuts are the only nuts that contain appreciable amounts of omega 3 fatty acids, which are anti-inflammatory. Walnuts help lower triglycerides and reduce plaque formation in arteries
- An excellent source of phosphorus, zinc, copper and thiamin and a good source of magnesium, iron, and potassium
- More than 70 percent of the fat comes from polyunsaturated fat.
- Rich in phytophenols and heart healthy antioxidants, known to lower cholesterol

SEEDS

Flax Seeds

- Flax seeds are the richest plant source of omega 3 fatty acids, which act as an anti-inflammatory and decrease blood levels of LDL cholesterol.
- High in fiber, calcium, and iron, flax seeds can boost nutrition levels when sprinkled on hot or cold cereal, pasta, and salad greens.
- Rich in lutein for eye health; lignans, and phytoestrogens help balance hormones in the body: flax also protects against breast cancer.

Pine Nuts

- The seeds of a variety of pine trees, including the North American piñon tree.

- Used to make pesto sauce; lightly toasted pine nuts are a great salad ingredient.
- They become rancid very easily and should be stored in the fridge or freezer.

Pumpkin/Squash Seeds

- In addition to its flesh, the seeds of a variety of winter squash are both tasty and nutritious. The most popular is the pumpkin seed.
- Pumpkin seeds are enclosed in a soft shell which is also edible for fiber. The seeds have a delicately nutty flavor.
- Pumpkin seeds are an excellent source of iron, phosphorus, potassium and zinc, and are high in protein and quite low in fat, a little less than half of which is polyunsaturated.

Safflower Seeds

- Common names for safflower seeds include safflower, false saffron, and saffron thistle.
- They are an excellent source of iron, magnesium, phosphorus, thiamin, and riboflavin and a good source of potassium and niacin.

Sesame Seeds

- Sesame seeds are tiny, with a paper-thin, edible hull. They may be white, yellow, brown, red, or black, and have a distinctive, nutty flavor.
- Sesame seeds are 40 to 60 percent oil by weight, most of which is polyunsaturated.
- They are an excellent source of calcium, iron, thiamin, riboflavin, and phosphorus and a good source of potassium.
- Sesame seeds are very versatile, used in breads and as a flavorful addition to baked goods. Sesame seed paste, tahini, is used in many dishes, e.g. hummus. Halvah, a sweet made from sesame seeds, is often found in health food shops.

Sunflower Seeds

- Colors of sunflower seeds can be grayish green, tan, or black. Shells are black and white striped.
- Sunflower seeds contain mostly polyunsaturated fat.
- Nutrients include vitamin E, folic acid, niacin, magnesium, potassium, selenium, and zinc.
- Sunflower seeds are high in plant sterols, particularly beta-sitosterol, known to lower blood cholesterol and good for prostate health.

Sources: usda.gov; Bowden, Jonny. *150 Healthiest Foods on Earth.* Fair Winds Press, 2007, and Pratt, Steven and Matthews, Kathy. *SuperFoods: 14 Foods that will Change Your Life.* HarperCollins. 2004;

NUTS AND SEEDS (1/2 CUP)	KCALS	PROTEIN (g)	FAT (g)	CARBS (g)	FIBER (g)	CALCIUM (mg)	IRON (mg)
Almonds	172	6	15	6	4	74	1
Beechnuts	172	2	15	10	0	0	1
Brazil nuts (Selenium 388 mcg)	133	3	13	2	2	32	0
Butternuts	145	6	14	3	1	13	1
Cashews	165	5	10	9	1	9	1
Chestnuts, Chinese (Vitamin A 202 IU)	224	4	1	49	0	18	1
Chestnuts, European	196	2	1	44	0	19	1
Coconut meat	125	1	12	5	3	5	1
Gingko nuts (Vitamin A 558 IU)	182	4	2	38	0	2	1
Hazelnuts or Filberts	155	4	15	4	2	28	1
Hickory nuts	155	3	15	4	2	14	1
Lotus seeds	89	4	1	17	0	44	1
Macadamia nuts	203	2	20	3	2	18	1
Peanut	170	8	15	4	3	17	.4
Pecans	179	2	19	4	3	18	1
Pine nuts	141	3	14	3	1	3	1
Pistachio nuts (Vitamin A 128 IU)	129	5	10	6	2	25	1
Pumpkin/Squash seeds (Zinc 5 mg)	198	8	9	24	0	24	1
Safflower seeds	109	3	8	7	0	16	1
Flaxseed (Lutien 110 mg)	90	3	7	5	5	43	1
Sesame seeds	113	3	10	5	2	192	3
Sunflower seeds	124	4	11	5	2	18	1
Walnuts, Black	140	5	13	2	2	14	1
Walnuts, English	158	4	16	3	2	24	1

MAGNESIUM (mg)	PHOSPHORUS (mg)	POTASSIUM (mg)	SODIUM (mg)	FOLATE (mcg)	SAT	MONO	POLY
82	141	217	0	9	8%	67%	25%
0	0	303	11	34	12%	46%	42%
76	147	133	1	4	25%	41%	34%
56	105	99	0	16	2%	19%	78%
54	101	117	3	14	21%	62%	18%
84	96	447	3	68	16%	56%	28%
30	38	484	2	58	20%	37%	43%
11	40	126	7	9	94%	5%	1%
27	124	510	7	54	21%	40%	40%
40	71	168	0	28	8%	79%	14%
41	79	103	0	9	11%	53%	36%
56	168	367	1	28	17%	21%	62%
28	40	78	1	2	17%	81%	2%
50	113	206	91	34	18%	52%	30%
31	72	106	0	6	9%	59%	32%
53	121	125	0	7	8%	33%	59%
28	113	237	0	12	13%	55%	32%
116	41	407	8	4	20%	33%	48%
74	135	144	1	34	10%	13%	77%
66	109	137	5	15	9%	19%	72%
69	124	92	2	19	15%	40%	46%
27	239	101	1	49	14%	16%	69%
46	116	119	0	7	6%	28%	66%
38	84	107	0	24	9%	14%	74%

18 Beans Are Best

Beans — including peas and lentils—are the best substitute for meat. They are filling, full of protein, fiber, and lots of other nutrients; they are versatile and easy to prepare once you know a few basics.

Tips for Adding Beans to Your Diet

- If you're really busy, buy beans canned. Because they can contain a lot of salt and can make your food sticky, rinse before using.
- Got a little time? Buy dried beans and soak overnight or 2 hours before cooking to avoid excess gas.
- Want to cut down on saturated fat? Mix beans with grains, especially rice and corn, for complete protein with less fat than meat (see suggestions below).
- Or mix beans with nuts and seeds, or grains for a high-quality complete protein. Remember succotash—limas and corn? A good example.
- Need more fiber? Beans have more fiber per serving than most other foods.
- Don't like beans? There are many different varieties and many imaginative uses, that might change your mind (see preparation tips below).
- Still don't like beans? Eat peas and lentils. They have similar nutrient profiles, but their taste and texture are quite different.

Benefits of Beans

- Beans have both soluble and insoluble fiber and no cholesterol.
- Beans are high in folate and other B vitamins, potassium, iron and magnesium.
- Beans have only 2-3% fat, low carbohydrates, and lots of protein.
- Beans help keep hunger at bay because they digest slowly and have complex carbs.

Nutrient Profiles per 1/2 cup (4 oz.) serving of cooked, drained beans

BEAN	CALORIES	PROTEIN (g)	FAT (g)	CARBS (g)	FIBER (g)	SUGGESTED USES
Adzuki beans	150	16.8	.18	28.5	8.4	Blend with rice & veggies; common in Asian dishes
Black beans	120	7.6	.28	23	4.9	Soups, stews, in salad with corn, rice, & beans
Black-eyed peas (cowbeans)	73	2.6	.35	16.5	4.1	Salads, casseroles, fritters, bean cakes; with ham in soups
Cannellini beans	120	8	.55	23	9.3	Soups, saute with greens, spreads & dips
Edamame (young soybeans)	94	8.5	4	7.7	4	In salads and stir frys
Fava beans (broad beans)	93	6.5	.35	16.6	4.5	Stews, & as a side dish
Garbanzo beans (chickpeas)	135	7.7	2.7	22.5	6.8	Hummus; minestrone; salads
Great Northern beans	170	11	.33	27	9	Soups, stew, saute with greens, spreads & dips
Green beans (includes pole beans)	25	2	.24	8.5	3.5	Side dish; soups; mix with nuts; salads; three bean salad
Kidney beans	110	18	.08	20.5	8.5	Chili, three bean salad, Cajun foods, stews
Lentils	113	9	.38	19.3	7.8	Soups; stews; with mixed vegetables; mashed with garlic
Lima beans (butter beans)	160	7.5	.65	25	6	Casseroles; succotash; soups, salads
Navy beans	125	7.5	.58	24	9.5	Soups, stews, chili, rice and beans
Peas, green	32	2.7	.2	5.2	2.3	Side dish, salads, soups, mixed with rice, pilafs, fried rice

BEAN	CALORIES	PROTEIN (g)	FAT (g)	CARBS (g)	FIBER (g)	SUGGESTED USES
Pinto beans	75	4.5	.25	15	4	Blend with rice, side dishes; filling for burritos, enchiladas, tacos
Soybeans	125	11	5.8	10	3.8	High protein; made into tofu, tempeh, miso, soy milk, etc.
Split peas	113	8.2	.4	20	8.2	Soups, blend with corn & lentils; serve with ham and bacon
White beans	120	8	.55	23	9.3	Soups, stews, with greens, spreads

Source: usda.gov/fnic/foodcomp

Cooking Tips

1. Rinse canned beans before use, unless you account for the extra sodium and starch in your recipe.
2. Buy dried beans from a source that has frequent turnover so you are sure they are fresh.
3. Soak beans before use to avoid excess gas and hasten cooking time.
   - *Overnight* - place 1 pound dried beans in 10 cups water. Cover and soak in refrigerator 6 to 8 hours or overnight. Rinse thoroughly before cooking.
   - *Quick soak* - bring 10 cups of water to a boil. Add 1 pound dried beans; return to a rolling boil and cook for 2 to 3 minutes; remove from heat, cover and let sit at room temperature for 1 hour. Rinse thoroughly before cooking.
   - *To minimize gas* caused by indigestible parts of beans, place 1 pound of beans in 10 or more cups of boiling water and bring to a rolling boil; cook for 3 minutes; cover and set aside overnight; indigestible fiber will dissolve into the water. Rinse beans twice, then cook.
4. Cover soaked beans with three times their volume of water. Add herbs or spices as desired (bay leaves, marjoram, celery, etc).

Bring to a boil, then simmer gently, uncovered, 45 minutes or until tender. Add more water as needed.

5. Wait until beans are almost done to add flavorings such as tomatoes, vinegar, and salt.
6. If cooked beans are to be stored for later use, immerse them in cold water to stop cooking; drain well and keep in refrigerator until use, or freeze.
7. One pound of dried beans yields about 5 or 6 cups cooked beans.
8. A 15-ounce can of beans equals about 1-1/2 cups cooked beans, drained.

Serving Tips

1. Add cooked beans to chili, tomato sauce, soup, salsa, or meat sauce as a main dish.
2. Blend with grains (esp. rice or corn); add a bit of salsa and hot sauce for a protein-rich side dish.
3. Make soup with beans as the main ingredient, or as a texture complement with vegetables.
4. Sauté garlic and onion in a bit of oil, add cooked beans and continue until heated. Add lemon juice and mash or process for a tasty vegetable dip or spread for crackers. Heart-healthy and protein-rich.
5. Sauté greens in a bit of oil and garlic and add beans. A great color and texture contrast.
6. Add corn to a three-bean salad for a high-quality complete protein.
7. Make a salad of corn, black beans, chopped onions, celery, and red peppers; dress with lemon juice, hot sauce, and bit of olive oil. Tasty, nutritious, and pretty.
8. There are many, many recipes and cooking tips on the Web. Check them out and enjoy.

19 Cooking & Seasoning Oils

BEST COOKING OILS	
Olive oil (extra virgin)	High in monounsaturated fatty acids and a fairly high smoke point for stir frying; many vareties available; most have a light, neutral flavor
Sunflower oil	Good balance of mono- and polyunsaturated fats and a source of omega 3 fatty acids; high smoke point
Peanut oil	Pale, fairly light oil neutral in flavor; cold pressed varieties easily available; good balance of mono- and polyunsaturated fats

BEST SEASONING OILS	
Sesame oil	Rich, aromatic flavor that pairs well with both meats and vegetables; can withstand fairly high heat
Walnut oil	Rich in omega 3 fatty acids, with a nutty flavor that goes well with vegetables, both raw and cooked
Avocado oil	High in monounsaturated fats; the faint, delicate flavor of aniseed goes well with fruit-based salads

*Choose only cold pressed varieties; heating destroys healthy nutrients.

Basics of Culinary Oils

- Oils for cooking and flavoring food are extracted from nuts and seeds, the fruits of plants. Oils provide nutrients from which the body makes essential fatty acids.
- Cooking oils are fairly neutral in flavor and withstand heat well. The more flavorful seasoning oils are used to season cold foods, and are added to hot foods at the last minute. They are used sparingly and often in combination with a neutral oil.
- Nutrient profiles of oils vary considerably, as shown below.
- Polyunsaturated fats vary also between types of fatty acids. For example, omega 3's are found in flaxseed oil and walnut oil. Soy, sesame, sunflower and corn oils have lots of omega-6's.

- Cold-pressed extra virgin oils have the least amount of processing and are the healthiest oils. (Heat destroys fragile nutrients.)
- Hydrogenated or partially hydrogenated oils are used to give a long shelf life to processed foods. They are very unhealthy and should be avoided.

(See "Nuts and Seeds" and "All About Fats")

Nutrient Profiles – Some Comparisons

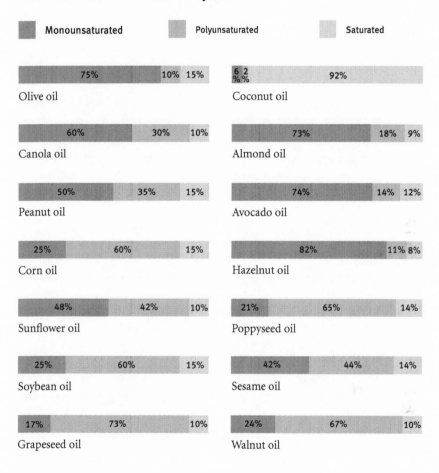

Monounsaturated   Polyunsaturated   Saturated

Oil	Monounsaturated	Polyunsaturated	Saturated
Olive oil	75%	10%	15%
Coconut oil	6%	2%	92%
Canola oil	60%	30%	10%
Almond oil	73%	18%	9%
Peanut oil	50%	35%	15%
Avocado oil	74%	14%	12%
Corn oil	25%	60%	15%
Hazelnut oil	82%	11%	8%
Sunflower oil	48%	42%	10%
Poppyseed oil	21%	65%	14%
Soybean oil	25%	60%	15%
Sesame oil	42%	44%	14%
Grapeseed oil	17%	73%	10%
Walnut oil	24%	67%	10%

COOKING OILS

Canola Oil

Also known as rapeseed oil, this neutral-flavored oil is suitable for frying, cooking, or baking. It has a high smoke point and is low in saturated fats. Because virtually all canola oil varieties are heat-processed, which destroys essential nutrients, many nutritionists do not recommend its use, even though it is high in monounsaturates.

Coconut Oil

Extracted from the dried kernel of the coconut, this is often used in commercial food preparations and in certain Indian dishes. It is high in saturated fats, but they are medium chain triglycerides (MCT) unlike the saturated fats from animals. One of them, lauric acid has been shown to be anti-microbial, anti-bacterial, and anti-viral, so it boosts immunity to a number of common infections. The saturated fats derived from plants seem to be neutral with respect to blood cholesterol, as long as they are not hydrogenated.

Corn Oil

One of the most economical and widely used all-purpose oils, this is deep yellow in color and heavy in texture. Corn oil is high in polyunsaturated fats and has a high smoke point, so it is ideal for most culinary preparations. Most common varieties are heat processed, which destroys essential nutrients. Because it is high in omega 6, use sparingly.

Cottonseed Oil

Derived from the cotton plant, this oil is used in the production of margarine and blended cooking oils. It is also used in Egyptian cuisine, where it lends a distinctive flavor. High in saturated fats, this oil is commonly used in processed foods, where it is heat processed and often hydrogenated. Not recommended for use in heart healthy diets.

Grapeseed Oil

A pale, delicate oil extracted from grape seeds, this product can withstand a wide range of temperatures. When refrigerated, it will not cloud, making it ideal for mayonnaise, and it has a very high smoke point, so it is excellent for frying and general cooking. It is high in polyunsaturated fats.

Macadamia Seed Oil

Considered by some to be the most healthful of cooking oils, it has even more monounsaturated fats than olive oil (85%), and its heart-healthy fatty acid profile raises HDLs and lowers triglycerides. It has a rich, nutty taste, good in a salad oil blend.

Olive Oil

There are as many different types and flavors of olive oil as wine, it seems. Depending on the species of tree, flavors can be neutral, grassy, earthy, pungent, or nutty. Rich in monounsaturated fats and with a high smoke point, olive oil is probably the healthiest and most versatile cooking oil you can use. It is full of antioxidant plant phenols. Extra virgin means it is the first pressing, and cold pressed means no heat is used in processing, both of which make the healthiest oil.

Red Palm Oil

Also known as palm nut oil or dende oil, this product is extracted from the pulp of the fruit of oil palms. Orange-gold in color, it has a pleasant nutty flavor. Although it is a general-purpose oil, being light in color and taste and good for frying and making salad dressings, it does, however, turn rancid very rapidly. Extra virgin, cold pressed palm oil is nothing like the hydrogenated type that is used in processed foods. It has a good balance of fats and is rich in antioxidant vitamin E and carotenoids.

Peanut Oil

This is a very fine, almost tasteless oil for general use in salads, cooking, and frying. The cold-pressed variety has a mild peanut flavor that is good with fruit-flavored vinegars for salad dressings. Peanut oil is moderately high in monounsaturates and low in saturates. Avoid heat processed varieties to get the best nutrient profile.

Safflower Oil

With a bright yellow color, this oil is ideal for all culinary uses, although the flavor is rather strong. Of all the cooking oils, peanut oil is one of the highest in polyunsaturated fats, lowest in saturated fats, and a good source of vitamin E.

Sesame Oil

There are many types of this oil. European, or cold-pressed sesame oil, is light in color and nutty in flavor with a high smoke point, making it a good cooking oil. Asian sesame oil is made from toasted sesame seeds, giving it a darker color and more pronounced taste. All are aromatic and capable of being heated to a high temperature and also used as a seasoning oil. Because it is high in omega 6's, some nutritionists discourage its use. But if you eat few processed foods, this is a good choice, at least in small quantities as a seasoning.

Soy Oil

A major component of blended oils, soy oil is a high-quality, neutral-flavored oil that is low in saturated fats. High in omega 6 fats, soy oil may not be the best choice for those who eat a lot of processed foots. Also, heat processing damages nutrients, so look for organic, cold pressed varieties.

Sunflower Oil

An all-purpose oil because of its neutral flavor, it is high in polyunsaturates, tasteless, pale, and light in texture. It can be used for frying, cooking, salad dressings, and mixing with other more strongly flavored oils. It has a good balance of mono- and polyunsaturated fats, but is high in omega 6's and may be heat processed.

Vegetable Oil

Vegetable oil is obtained from blending a number of oils in various proportions, and types and quantities are not necessarily given on the label. It may contain coconut or palm oils, which are high in saturated fats. Vegetable oil has little aroma or flavor, making it popular as an all-purpose culinary oil.

SEASONING OILS

Almond Oil

A pale oil made from sweet almonds, almond oil is used in baking and confectionery. Use to coat cake pans or cookie sheets when preparing delicate baked goods, or heat gently with slivered almonds and serve with fish or cooked green vegetables. It is high in monounsaturated fat, like olive oil, and has a high smoke point, so it can also be used for cooking.

Avocado Oil

Extracted from the pits of avocados and sometimes from blemished fruit, this oil is colorless with a faint aniseed flavor. It is unusually high in monounsaturated fats, making it exceptionally heart healthy. Its delicate flavor pairs well other oils to dress fruit-based salads.

Flaxseed Oil

Made from flax seeds, one of only three oils (also hemp and walnut oils) that has omega-3 fats which can't be made by the body. Flax is rich in lignans, which protect against hormone-sensitive cancers, like breast, uterine, and prostate. Use it in salad dressing, blended with more flavorful olive oil, or take as a supplement.

Hazelnut Oil

This oil is a delicious, richly flavored oil, best used with light vinegars for salad dressings or as a marinade for fish or poultry. Unusually high in monounsaturated fats, it is exceptionally heart healthy. Heating destroys nutrients and flavor. Sprinkle onto meat or vegetables at the last minute or into sauces that have cooled slightly. It can be used for baking sweet, nutty pastries.

Hemp Seed Oil

Like flax, hemp seeds and oil have an excellent balance between types of fats, and between omega 3's and omega 6's. Its fatty acids lower LDL cholesterol and improve insulin sensitivity. Hemp seed oil should not be heated, but can be blended with other flavoring oils to boost their nutrient profile. It has a nutty, grainy flavor that is good in salad dressings. Look for organic oil that has been cold pressed.

Pine Seed Oil

With a distinctive pine seed flavor, this oil is produced on small European farms for a gourmet cooking market. Add small amounts to veggie dips, salad dressings and sauces for an unusual taste treat.

Pumpkin Seed Oil

This oil is dark brown with a pleasant flavor of toasted pumpkin seeds. Do not heat, but use in dipping sauces or as a last-minute seasoning for steamed vegetables or fish.

Walnut Oil

A delicious topaz-colored oil with a rich, nutty flavor. Walnut oil does not keep long, either opened or unopened, so buy in small quantities and keep in a cool place, but not in the refrigerator. It makes delicious salad dressings and dipping sauces. It is also good with fish, poultry, and vegetables and can be used in baking sweet pastries when a walnut flavor is desired.

Source: usda.gov; Adapted from: Bowden, Jonny. *150 Healthiest Foods on Earth.* Fair Winds Press. 2007 and http://www.theepicentre.com/tip/nutandseedoils.html

20 Twenty-five Low-Carb Fruits and Vegetables

- The number of calories in fruits and vegetables depends on how much sugar and starch they have, compared to water and fiber.
- Sugar and starch are carbs, which have 4 calories per gram. Fiber and water provide no calories. Therefore, the more water and fiber in a serving, and fewer carbs, the lower the calories.
- The volume (cups) of fruits and vegetables is not relevant. You can have ½ cup of lettuce with 10 calories and the same ½ cup of mashed potatoes for 100 calories. Potatoes weigh a lot more than lettuce and have a lot more carbs!

Here is a list of fruits and vegetables from lowest to highest calories *per 50 grams*. You can assume that most of the difference between the grams of carbs and 50 grams is water, which has no calories. So, the more watery the food, the fewer calories it will have by weight.

VEGGIES (50 GRAMS)	GRAMS OF CARBS	TOTAL CALORIES
Arugala	1	13
Cucumber	1	6
Broccoli Rabe	1	17
Lettuce	2	7
Celery	2	8
Mushrooms	2	11
Radishes	2	21
Turnips	2	20
Romaine	2	10
Asparagus	2	10
Sweet pepper (green)	2	10
Okra	2	19
Cauliflower	3	13
Sweet pepper (yellow)	3	15
Cabbage	3	13
Sweet pepper (red)	3	15

Sources: dlife.com; usda.gov

VEGGIES (50 GRAMS)	GRAMS OF CARBS	TOTAL CALORIES
Broccoli	4	17
Spinach	4	16
Beets	4	22
Green Beans	4	16
Carrot	5	21
Kale	5	23
Sugar Snap Peas	5	21
Onions	7	28
Sweet Corn	10	54

Sources: dlife.com; usda.gov

FRUITS (50 GRAMS)	GRAMS OF CARBS	TOTAL CALORIES
Watermelon	4	15
Strawberries	4	16
Cantaloupe	4	17
Avocado	4	80
Honeydew	5	20
Peach	5	20
Blackberries	5	21
Grapefruit	5	24
Orange	5	24
Papaya	5	20
Nectarine	6	24
Clementine	6	27
Plums	6	24
Raspberries	6	26
Pineapple	6	25
Blueberries	7	28
Apple	7	28
Pear	7	29
Kiwi Fruit	8	32
Tangerine	8	32
Cherries	8	32
Mango	8	32
Persimmon	9	36
Banana	12	48
Grapes	13	35

Sources: dlife.com; usda.gov

21 Unfamiliar Foods You Might Like To Try

Artichokes	(French globe) – looks like a large green pine cone with thorns on top of its leaves, but don't let looks deceive you. Artichokes are delicious, both leaves and hearts, if you know how to cook and eat them. Cut off the stem and bottom of the choke. Then simply simmer in salted water until the color has become muted (about 30 minutes). Pull out one leaf to see if it is done. If it pulls out with just a slight tug, it is ready. Pull out the leaves and use your front teeth to scrape the flesh off the bottom. Dipping the ends of the leaves in melted butter is optional. When all the leaves are gone, scrape off the fuzz on top of the heart, cut off the top ¼ inch of the heart, and quarter the heart. It is delicious on its own, or with butter. Practice helps.
	Low in calories, artichokes are one of the richest plants in protein and are chock full of vitamins and minerals and phytochemicals (Vitamins A, B1-3, and C; calcium, magnesium, iron, potassium, and zinc) and a huge amount of fiber. They are worth the work it takes to eat them
Bok Choy	Also known as Chinese cabbage. Like most leafy vegetables, bok choy is very low in calories, but high in nutrients; it is rich in Vitamins A, C, and K, choline, calcium, potassium, and folate. Just slice it in chunks and add to stir-fry or soups at the last minute. Because it cooks very quickly, it will lose its crispness if cooked more than a couple of minutes. Buckets of beta carotene.
Dandelion leaves	Dandelion has a long history as one of the best health-promoting remedies. Its phytochemicals are known to detoxify the liver and stimulate digestion. On top of that, it is a piquant addition to salad greens, adding a spicy, slightly bitter taste.
	Dandelion scores near the top of all vegetables for beta-carotene, bone and blood-building Vitamin K, and the third richest source of Vitamin A and minerals that support eye health. A nutritional powerhouse!
Endive	Another leafy vegetable low in calories. Eat it raw in salad or cooked in stir-fry or soup. Stuffed with goat cheese and colorful chopped veggies like beets or peppers, it makes a great appetizer. For very few calories, it is stuffed with Vitamins A and K, choline, potassium, and manganese. Full of beta-carotene.
Herring	This little fish is most frequently found in jars in the dairy sec-

tion in cream sauce with onions or in a light wine sauce. Both are delicious. The fish are firm and their taste is not too fishy. They make great appetizers. In addition to being a rich source of complete protein, herring is exceedingly rich in vital omega 3's and selenium.

Jicama	A root vegetable grown mostly in Mexico, jicama is a staple of Mexican cooking. Its skin looks like a potato, and it's shaped like a large onion, but it is nothing like either. The closest I can come to describing its flesh is a water chestnut, though it is less starchy and sweeter.
	Jicama is great raw on a veggie tray or in salad, and cooked in stir fry and soup. It is low calorie and rich in Vitamin C, fiber, and potassium and modest amounts of calcium and magnesium.
Kohlrabi	Kohlrabi looks like a pale green turnip with three or four long stems ending in broad leaves The leaves and stems are a great addition to soups. The round bottom can be eaten raw like an apple, or sliced into soups, or boiled and mashed like potatoes. In fact, a gourmet dish which is half mashed kohlrabi and half mashed potatoes is delicious and served in some of the best restaurants.
	Kohlrabi is an excellent source of Vitamin C, potassium, and phosphorus, buts its main value is in cancer-fighting phytochemicals and a whopping amount of fiber (5 g per serving).
Miso	A staple of the Japanese diet, miso is a thick paste made of fermented soybeans. It takes only a little to make a nice light soup as a healthy meal starter. Or use a bit in other soups, stews or casseroles as a nutrition and flavor enhancer. It offers a good serving of protein and is rich in selenium, potassium, phosphorus and almost 4 g of fiber in just ½ cup.
	Health alert: Miso has lots of sodium, so use with caution if you need to restrict sodium. If sodium is well balanced with potassium, it is usually not a problem in the same way sodium chloride (salt) can be. But check with your health care provider to make sure miso is a good choice for you.
Okra	One of the oddest looking vegetables, okra is a green tubular pod full of seeds. Fried or boiled, it has long been a staple of southern cooking, but is fairly unknown in the North. It is often sliced into soups, particularly gumbo, or served with cooked tomatoes as a side dish.
	Full of fiber, vitamins and minerals, okra packs a nutritional punch, particularly because it is surprisingly low in calories. It can be found frozen in many supermarkets and fresh in season.

	Okra is a great source of Vitamins C and K and rich in calcium, magnesium, potassium, folate, and manganese.
Oysters	For the squeamish, oysters don't have to be eaten raw, though some find oysters a coveted delicacy. Oysters can be used in soups and stews, and smoked oysters in sardine-size cans have an entirely different, sweet taste which is excellent on crackers with a bit of cream cheese or goat cheese. Oysters are a top choice for Vitamin B12 and the important minerals zinc, copper, iron, and chromium.
Papaya	Papaya is a tropical fruit that looks like a large, elongated green and yellow mango. It has red flesh similar to a watermelon, but is sweeter and less watery. Low in calories, it is full of beta carotenes and other antioxidants, as well as Vitamin A and C and potassium.
Parsnips	Parsnips look like white carrots, but they are related to turnips, with most of the same properties. Best cooked in stir fries or added to soups, parsnips are also delicious mashed by themselves or with mashed potatoes.
Quinoa	Pronounced "keen-wah," quinoa is one of the healthiest foods you can eat. Quinoa is not technically a grain, but related to beets and Swiss chard. Its seeds are eaten like a grain, often as a substitute for rice. It cooks rapidly, the seeds swelling to 3 or 4 times their dry size. Quinoa has more protein, minerals, B vitamins, and unsaturated fat, and less carbohydrate, than rice, and has a chewy texture. It's full of both soluble and insoluble fiber and has a whopping 4 mg of iron per serving. Rinse quinoa well before cooking. Raw quinoa may be coated with saponin, which can leave a bitter, soapy taste. Eat it alone, or in soups, casseroles, or even hot for breakfast.
Sardines	Sardines are not actually that unusual and have long been a favorite staple in the American diet. But recently the power-packed little fish have fallen out of favor, which is too bad because they are one of the most nutrient-rich foods we could eat. Not only are they a rich source of protein and Vitamin B12, but they offer unequaled amounts of essential omega 3's. Sardines are great in salads, on sandwiches, and as rich, tasty appetizers.
Sauerkraut	Sauerkraut is found in many deli sandwiches, of course, but is rarely found in modern kitchens along with more popular vegetables. It is shredded cabbage which has been fermented and cooked.
	Sauerkraut has the same very healthful nutrient profile particular to fermented foods like miso and kim-chi, a staple of Korean

cooking. Low in calories, it is rich in vitamin K and potassium, but is also high in sodium.

Water Chestnuts	Water chestnuts, those toothsome little round white morsels so familiar in oriental dishes, have lots of other uses. Dice them and add to tuna salad or pasta salad for an unexpected crunch. Or slice and add to a green salad for a color and texture surprise.
Watercress	This tender green leafy vegetable packs a surprising nutritional punch. It is loaded with Vitamins A, B1, B2, B6, C, K, manganese, potassium, sodium, and so many phytochemicals it is off the charts. In sandwiches or salads, it has a slight peppery flavor that adds lots of zing. It may be hard to find, but pester your produce department to get it because a little goes a long way, nutritionally speaking.
Wheat germ	Wheat germ is the nutrient-rich "seed" of a whole wheat kernel, after the husk, bran, and endosperm have been removed. Rich in protein, it also offers vitamin E, zinc, iron, fiber, folic acid, chromium, magnesium, and a host of other trace minerals. A couple of tablespoons is all you need, sprinkled on cereal or salad, or added to soups, stews, or casserole toppings.

22 Spices and Herbs

Cooks have been experimenting with spices and herbs for thousands of years. You can benefit from all that experience by learning just a few simple cooking techniques and a few food and seasoning combinations. Once you do, you'll lose interest in bland prepared foods and love your own cooking.

SPICES are dried seeds, fruits, roots, or bark of the plant. Spices will last for several months if kept in a cool, dry place, but should be replaced regularly, at least once a year.

HERBS are the leaves and stems of plants. Many herbs are available as both fresh and dried leaves. Dried leaves have concentrated flavor, so you use about 1/3 of what you would use fresh. Dried herbs keep in a cool, dark place, but after several months should be replaced.

Researchers are discovering more and more **HEALTH BENEFITS** of spices and herbs. The leaves of many herbs have amounts of antioxidants that rival antioxidant-rich fruits like blueberries. One half teaspoon of ground cinnamon has as much as a half cup of blueberries, and dried oregano has more antioxidants per serving than spinach. Mixing a bit of oregano, rosemary, ginger, and black pepper into ground beef results in much less carcinogens when the meat is grilled.

Tips for Using Spices and Herbs

1. If you don't smell a significant aroma when you open a bottle of spices or herbs, replace it. Most spices and herbs are highly aromatic.
2. Crushing spices and herbs just before using enhances the flavor addition to your dish. (You can invest in a mortar and pestle, but the back of a sturdy spoon will usually do just fine. Dry herbs can be rolled between your palms to gently crush them.)

3. Add about half of what the recipe (or your instincts) call for at first, tasting as you add a little more at a time. Same goes for salt.
4. A pinch of sugar in a quart of tomato-based dishes brings out the flavor.
5. Use savory spices in place of salt if you need to watch your sodium intake.

Here is a list of spices and herbs most commonly used in typical U.S. cooking and some popular ethnic cooking.

Meats & Vegetables (broiled, roasted, soups, stews, casseroles

Allspice	Fennel	Sage
Aniseed	Garlic	Savory
Bay leaves	Marjoram	Tarragon
Cloves	Rosemary	

Creamed, cheesy, or egg dishes (soups, sauces, dips)

Bay leaves	Chives	Nutmeg
Chervil	Garlic	

Tomato-based dishes (spaghetti sauce, pizza)

Basil	Ginger	Tarragon
Chervil	Saffron	Thyme

Fish, seafood, eggs

Basil	Marjoram	Tarragon
Cilantro	Oregano	Thyme

Pickled vegetables

Caraway	Dill

Hot dishes (chili, barbecue, curry)

Cayenne	Cumin	Turmeric
Chili flakes	Paprika	

Salads & Dressings

Basil	Garlic	Thyme
Dill weed	Savory	Turmeric
Dill seed		

Baked goods (breads, cookies, pastries, cakes, muffins) and fruit

Allspice	Coriander	Mint
Aniseed	Ginger	Nutmeg
Cardamom	Mace	Vanilla
Cloves		

Common Spices and Herbs

Allspice	Berries are dark brown balls just a little larger than peppercorns, dried and ground; used in pickling spices, spiced tea mixes, cakes, cookies, and pies. Food producers use it in ketchup, pickles, and sausages. Also used in Jamaican jerk seasoning for soups, stews, and curries.
Aniseed	Aniseed, sometimes spelled as anise, has a sweet licorice-like taste; whole or ground seeds are usually used in breads, a number of desserts, and quite often in savory dishes like Indian curries, mole, and a variety of fish and meat dishes, pickles, stews, seafood, beets, cauliflower and pasta sauces.
Basil	The aromatic, leafy flavor and aroma of basil is most intense during the summer months, when fresh basil is abundant. Used to flavor tomato dishes and tomato paste and spaghetti sauces; also used in cooking peas, squash, snap beans; sprinkle chopped over lamb chops and poultry. The oils in basil are highly volatile; it is best to add near the end of the cooking process.
Bay Leaves	The dried leaves of an evergreen grown in the eastern Mediterranean countries, basil has a sweet, herbaceous floral spice note. For pickling, stews, for spicing sauces and soup. Also use with a variety of meats and fish, especially soups and stews. Sometimes used as a spice in breads, especially rye bread.
Caraway Seeds	Small dark seeds with a flavor of anise and dill; used in rye breads; often added to sauerkraut, noodles, cheese spreads, potatoes, liver and canned asparagus
Cardamom	Traditionally used in curry blends, and as a flavoring for coffee, specialty breads, and apple pie
Cayenne Pepper	A hot, red chili pepper used to flavor dishes and for medicinal purposes. The fruits are generally dried and ground to make the powdered spice known as cayenne pepper; excellent added to cheese dishes and creamy sauces and soups.
Chervil	Available as fresh leaves or dried and crushed. Fresh chervil has a hint of anise and dry has a hint of parsley; goes well with fish, scrambled eggs and omelets, poultry, cream cheese and herb sandwiches, salads and even mashed potatoes.
Chili Flakes	Chili flakes are the dried seeds of chili pods, which are the hottest parts of a chili. The amount of heat in chili flakes depends on the variety of chili pepper and where it was grown. Crushed dried red chilies can be added to or sprinkled over all kinds of dishes for an extra kick; can be used in salad dressings, marinades and to spice up your favorite sauté.

Chives	The smallest member of the onion family with a mild onion flavor. Available as fresh or freeze-dried hollow stems. Delicate and peppery, chives are sprinkled on food just before serving. Use for potatoes, eggs, sauces, seafood and salads.
Cilantro	Wide delicate lacy green leaves and a pungent flavor; use for salsa, tomatoes, chicken, pork and seafood. The seed of the cilantro plant is known as coriander.
Cinnamon	A sweet spice widely used in many cultures; commonly used in cakes and other baked goods, milk and rice puddings, chocolate dishes and fruit desserts, particularly apples and pears. Also used in curries and garam masala, a spice mixture from India; available in sticks and ground into powder.
Cloves	Available whole or ground, these dried flower buds are used in savory and sweet dishes. Cloves can easily overpower a dish, particularly when ground, so use sparingly. A bit sprinkled in cooked grains adds a pungent flavor; often used to flavor ham and pork, and game meats, especially venison, wild boar and hare.
Coriander	Ground seeds are traditional in desserts and sweet pastries as well as in curries, meat, and seafood dishes; a highly aromatic spice, it's delicious with most meats, particularly lamb.
Cumin	This warm, pungent spice is the small dried fruit of a plant in the parsley family; one of the main ingredients in curry powder, it goes well with beans, chicken, couscous, eggplant, fish, lamb, lentils, peas, pork, potatoes, rice, sausages, soups, stews, eggs.
Dill Seed	The small dark seed of the dill plant has a grassy, aromatic taste; fresh and dried leaves flavor foods, such as gravlax (cured salmon), borscht and pickles; freeze-dried dill leaves stay flavorful for a few months and add a pleasing flavor to sauerkraut, potato salad, cooked macaroni, and green apple pie. Seeds go well in salad dressings and sauces and dips for vegetables.
Dill Weed	Dill seed and weed come from the same plant, but they do not substitute for each other. The seed is slightly bitter and aromatic, and dill weed has a subtle, grassy scent and taste. It pairs well with all kinds of seafood, egg-based casseroles and omelets, and white boiled potatoes.
Fennel Seeds	These little green seeds have a sweet, aniseed-like flavor that goes well with chicken and fish; it's the familiar flavor in Italian sausage and some curry powder mixes. Toasting seeds accentuates their flavor; fresh fennel is often used in salads or blanched and tossed into stir-fries.

Garlic	Fresh, dried and powdered garlic are available everywhere. Under a papery skin are segments called cloves, which are peeled, then chopped or minced. The flavor is distinctive--somewhat hot and pungent when raw, it becomes mild and sweet when cooked. A staple flavor for a wide variety of meat and vegetable dishes, sauces, dressings, marinades, and dips.
Ginger	The underground stem of the ginger plant. Used in almost every cooking culture, it doubles as sweet and savory. Common in stir fries, baked goods, beverages, and seafood.
Mace	The bright red, lacy covering of the nutmeg seed shell; similar to nutmeg but stronger. A light powder, it can substitute for nutmeg to avoid dark flakes, as in cream sauces and light pastries.. Add a bit to hot chocolate to punch up the flavor.
Marjoram	A member of the mint family, but similar to oregano; has a mild, fragrant, flavor sweeter than oregano with perhaps a hint of balsam. Considered the best herb for meat dishes, but good on vegetables and eggs as well.
Mint	Mint leaves have a pleasant warm, fresh, aromatic, sweet flavor with a cool aftertaste; used in teas, beverages, jellies, syrups, candies, and ice creams.
Mustard Seed	Available ground or as seeds; pungent, sharp, hot flavor. Use for meats, vinaigrettes, seafood and sauces.
Nutmeg	Nutmeg is the whole or ground seed of an evergreen; commonly used with fruits and sweet vegetables; also good in cheese sauces and is best grated fresh; traditional ingredient in mulled cider and wine, and sprinkled on eggnog.
Oregano	Dried leaves of the oregano plant; widely used in tomato sauces, fried vegetables, and grilled meats; combines nicely with pickles, olives, and capers. also works with hot and spicy food; most closely associated with pizza.
Paprika	Made from grinding dried capsicum (e.g. bell peppers). Used to season and color rice, stews, sausage and and soups; smoked paprika is a key ingredient in chorizo.
Parsley	Available year round as fresh leaves, curly or Italian (flat leaf), or dried and flaked. Commonly used as a garnish. Fresh parsley has a slightly peppery flavor; you can chop and freeze parsley; use for poultry, seafood, tomatoes, pasta, soups, and vegetables.
Pepper	A berry grown in grapelike clusters on the pepper plant; three basic types: black, white, and green; available whole, cracked, and ground. Can be used on virtually any non-sweet food: cheese, eggs, fish, meats, salad, sausages, soup, tomatoes.

Poppy Seeds	Fragrant and crunchy, with a nut-like flavor. Excellent as a topping for breads, rolls and cookies. Also delicious in buttered noodles and sweet vegetables.
Rosemary	A woody herb with fragrant needle-like leaves. Fresh and dried leaves have a bitter, astringent taste, which complements a wide variety of foods, especially lamb dishes, soups, and stews. Sprinkle on beef before roasting.
Saffron	The dried stigmas of the saffron crocus. Available as threads (whole stigmas) or powder. Pungent, intense, bitter flavor. Distinctive color makes rice yellow; combines well with fish and seafood, use for bouillabaisse, curries, fish, poultry and rice. Use sparingly.
Sage	Has large, slightly furry leaves when fresh; has a very strong, peppery-tasting flavor; use sparingly. Dried sage goes particularly well with pork or in pasta sauces and in stuffings. Great for meat and poultry stuffing, sausages, meat loaf, hamburgers, stews and salads.
Savory	A bold, peppery flavor, reminiscent of mint and thyme; available as fresh leaves, dried and crushed or ground. The leaves dry and keep well and blend easily with other herbs; use in stews, vegetable dishes, pizza toppings, and as a seasoning for roasting beef and fish. Also good with beans, lentils, lamb and poultry.
Sesame Seeds	Sesame seeds add a sweet nutty taste and crunch to many meat and vegetable dishes; the main ingredient in tahini, a paste used as a flavoring in sauces and dips; use in stir fries and sprinkle on steamed vegetables, seafood, noodles, and salads. Toasting enhances their flavor.
Tarragon	A fragrant herb with a strong aniseed flavor; most often used in fish and chicken dishes. used as a flavoring for vinegar and pickles, relishes, prepared mustards, and sauces; goes well with fish, meat, soups and stews, and is often used in tomato and egg dishes.
Thyme	The leaves are stems of a shrub with a strong aroma and distinctive flavor, which complements beans, eggs and vegetable dishes; in either its fresh or dried form, it should be added toward the end of the cooking process since heat can easily cause a loss of its delicate flavor. Great in pasta sauce, soup stocks, omelets and scrambled eggs. Poach fish with some sprigs in the poaching liquid.

Turmeric	A root of the ginger family, turmeric has a peppery, warm and bitter flavor and a mild fragrance similar to orange and ginger; one of the ingredients in curry powder and gives ballpark mustard its bright yellow color; use as a flavoring in dressings and salads.
Vanilla	Dried vanilla pods (beans) are long and black, encasing hundreds of tiny black seeds. Natural liquid vanilla extract is distilled from vanilla pods. Use with cooked apples and apricots, add to chocolate and custards.

Common Spice Blends

Chili powder (Mexico)	Contains paprika, cumin, coriander, nutmeg, ginger, black pepper, star anise, cardamom, cloves, mustard grains, saffron
Curry powder (India)	There are many different brands with varying blends, but it is usually a blend of up to 20 different herbs and spices, including cardamom, chilies, cinnamon, cloves, coriander, cumin, fennel, fenugreek, mace, nutmeg, pepper, poppy seeds, sesame seeds, saffron, tamarind and turmeric (which gives curry its characteristic golden color). Some recipes also contain ginger, garlic, asafoetida, fennel seed, caraway, mustard seed, green cardamom, black cardamom.
Five-spice powder (China)	A mixture of ground spices, including anise, pepper, cassia, fennel seeds, star anise and cloves. Use sparingly—it is pungent. Contrasting flavors—sweet, warm, cool and spicy—complement, rice, vegetables, pork and virtually any type of stir fry. A tiny amount adds mystery to muffins, nut breads, or even waffle batter.
Four-spice powder (France)	Contains ground pepper (white, black, or both), cloves, nutmeg and ginger. Some variations of the mix use allspice instead of pepper, or cinnamon in place of ginger.
Garam masala (India)	This mixture of ground roasted spices is made from cumin, coriander, cardamom and black pepper and is used in many Asian dishes.
Herbs de Provence (France)	A blend of savory, fennel, basil, thyme, and lavender.
Poultry seasoning (USA)	Made up of parsley, rosemary, sage, onion powder and thyme,
Pumpkin pie spices (USA)	Contains powdered cinnamon, cloves, ginger, nutmeg, and sometimes allspice.

List adapted from: www.realfood4realpeople.com/spice.html

PART 2

Choosing Which Foods To Eat

SOME THINGS TO CONSIDER

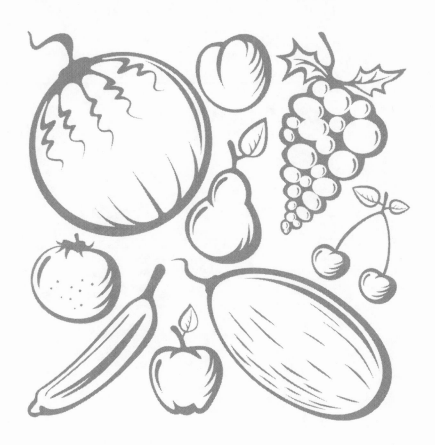

23 Food Comparisons

Meat, Dairy & Oils – Carbs & Fats Compared

LO FAT HI CARB ↑	Non fat dairy products (milk, cream, cottage cheese, yogurt, sour cream) Low fat dairy products (milk, cream, cottage cheese, yogurt, sour cream) Buttermilk Legumes (beans, lentils, peas) Soy milk/cheese/tofu Lean meat, poultry, fish	Non fat cheeses Non fat creams Eggs Nuts and seeds Olives Nuts and seed oils	LO FAT HI CARB ↑
↓ HI FAT LO CARB	Whole fat dairy products (milk, yogurt, cottage cheese, sour cream) High fat meat, poultry w/ skin	Olive oil Avocado Butter Full fat cheeses	↓ HI FAT LO CARB

Grains, Fruits & Vegetables – Carbs & Fiber Compared

HI FIBER LO CARB ↑	Grain brans (wheat, flax) Whole grains (wheat, rice, rye, barley) Moderately processed grains (brown rice, grits, oatmeal, wild rice, whole grain flours, whole wheat pasta)	High cellulose fruits & veggies (celery, broccoli, cabbage) High water fruits & veggies (melons, berries, cucumbers, summer squash) Leafy green vegetables (spinach, kale, lettuce, collards) Legumes (beans, lentils, peas) Thin or no skin fruits (apples, apricots, plums, peaches, grapefruit) Thin or no skin vegetables (potatoes, winter squash) High sugar fruits and veggies	HI FIBER LO CARB ↑
↓ LO FIBER HI CARB	Highly processed grains (white flour, white rice, pasta, cereals, breads, crackers, pastries)	Fruit and vegetable juice Wine and some beers Sugar, honey, syrup, corn syrup	↓ LO FIBER HI CARB

Prepared ("Ready to eat") Foods

	MOSTLY PROTEIN FOODS	MOSTLY CARBOHYDRATE FOODS	MOSTLY FAT FOODS
LO FAT LO CARB	Non fat cheese Non fat cream Non fat non dairy creamer Canned fish in water	Frozen green veggies (spinach, green beans) Frozen fruits, popsicles Popcorn without butter Dark chocolate	

LO FAT HI CARB	Non fat ice cream
	Lo fat ice cream
	
	Spaghetti
	Most canned sauces/mixes
	Most "lean" frozen
	  entrees/dinners
	Power bars
		Bread
		Packaged mixes
		  (bread, cakes, rolls, stuffing)
		Frozen fruit juices
		Frozen high starch veggies
		  (potatoes, peas, corn, limas)
		Cereals
		Crackers
		Cookies
		Fruit pies
		Sherbet/Sorbet
		Soda pop
		Pretzels
		Rice crackers
		Most hard candy	

HI FAT LO CARB	Canned meat, poultry, fish
	Fast food chicken
	Frozen fried chicken & fish
	Power bars
		Commercial peanut butter
		Cheesy snacks
		Fast food salads
			Flavored
			  salad
			  dressings
			Mayonnaise
			Margarine
			Nuts

HI FAT HI CARB	Egg nog
	Premium ice cream and
	  toppings
	Custards
	Fast food burgers, tacos, etc.
	Most frozen entrees
	  (fried meats and fish,
	  egg rolls, pizza)
	Most frozen dinners
	Most canned entrees
		Pizza (cheese)
		Popcorn w/oil and/or butter
		Frozen veggies in cream sauce
		Frozen fried veggies
		French fries
		Potato chips
		Doughnuts
		Waffles
		Cream pies
		Most cream, nut, and/or
		  chocolate candies	

24 Nutrient Density

1. Nutrient density is a measure of how much nutritional bang you are getting for your calorie buck.
2. Most foods have both
   A. energy value (calories provided by carbs, proteins, and fats) and
   B. nutritional value (no-calorie vitamins, minerals, and phytochemicals such as antioxidants).
3. Calories provide energy for daily activities and for building tissues.
4. Vitamins, minerals, and phytochemicals enable the body to fulfill its normal functions.
5. The nutritional value of a food relative to its calorie value is its nutrient density—essentially the ratio of nutrients to calories. The higher the nutrient/calorie ratio, the better.
   A. For example, say you have a cup of peas and a cup of vanilla pudding, both having approximately 200 calories. The cup of peas has many more vitamins, minerals, phytochemicals, and fiber than the cup of vanilla pudding. Therefore, its nutrient density is greater.
   B. If you have two cups of leafy green vegetables and a quarter cup of white rice, they both have about 50 calories. But the nutrients in the 50 calories of leafy greens are much higher than the nutrients in 50 calories of white rice. Therefore, the nutrient density of the greens is higher than the rice, even though they are both are reasonably good for you.

Here's a summary of how to choose healthful, nutrient-dense foods as often as possible:

First – fresh or frozen veggies and fruit – eat all you want

Because they are low in calories and high in nutrients, vegetables and fruits generally have the highest nutrient value per calorie of all foods, and dark green leafy veggies have the most of all. So the more colorful vegetables and fruit you eat, the better your diet. Starchy vegetables and some fruits, while high in nutrients, are also high in calories, so you could eat those more moderately, especially if you are watching your weight.

Second – beans (legumes), nuts and seeds, and whole grains – eat in moderation

Few of us want to restrict our food to just vegetables and fruit. So the next best category of food is beans, seeds and nuts, and whole grains. They are higher in calories, but are such nutritional powerhouses that the calories are really worth it. And the mix of legumes and grains provides all essential amino acids (protein).

Third – dairy, fish, eggs – eat in moderation

Many vegetarians allow a moderate amount of dairy and eggs in their diets. This is a good choice, because they are a good source of complete protein and have a fairly good nutrient to calorie ratio.

Fourth – cheese, butter, meat, vegetable oils, margarine, mayonnaise – eat modest amounts, or as a flavoring or as a treat

Vegetable oils are an essential ingredient in a healthy diet, and have important nutrients to balance the high calories. Meat and cheese are good sources of complete protein and essential nutrients. Butter and mayonnaise are most often used as flavorings or condiments. There are good reasons to eat these high calorie foods; just do it sparingly, occasionally, and wisely.

Fifth– refined grains (bread, pasta), highly processed foods in cans or boxes, prepared foods (pizza, take out and fast food), and sweets – eat as infrequently as possible

While eating whole grains and fresh food cooked at home is the ideal, it's not always convenient or possible, given Americans' typical work and social lives. If you consciously try to seek vegetables when you eat out and whole grains when you can, eating the occasional hot dog or pizza is not unreasonable. Sweets such as ice cream and pastries are generally empty calories, but are reasonable treats. Chocolate is full of empty calories, to be sure, but also has some really good nutrition.

25 Serving Sizes and Portion Control

Serving Sizes

- How much is a serving of vegetables?
- Who decides what a serving is on nutrition labels? The manufacturer? The government?
- If I want to count calories, do I have to weigh and measure everything I eat?
- Where can I find out what one "standard" serving is?

Try putting your usual serving of cooked pasta on a plate, then put it in a measuring cup. Chances are your serving will be considerably larger than the government's "standard" of ¾ cup. Or compare your baked potato to the average size of a "medium" potato (a computer mouse) as recommended by the USDA's MyPyramid program. It's likely to be double the size, in part because growers have bred potatoes to be larger than "average" to increase their yields.

Anyone who tries to follow government recommendations for healthy eating, or for following a diet, or simply for limiting the number of calories she or he eats runs into the problem of "how much?"

The U.S. Department of Agriculture has tried to solve the problem by establishing standard serving sizes and using those standards to form the basis of their recommendations for the MyPyramid program, which requires specific numbers of servings per day or per week for each food group.

Actual eating is not so simple. Portions of prepared foods are usually much larger than any standard serving sizes; restaurant servings range from miniscule to huge; frozen entrees seem tiny by comparison—many people eat two for one meal.

We are so used to eating food prepared by someone else, where serving size is determined by commercial motives, many of us overestimate by double or even triple what a standard serving size really is. Manufacturers and restaurants are not required to establish their serving sizes to conform to government standards.

Portion Control

Visualizing portions is easy, quick, and works in all situations. You can use it to count servings, and even approximate calories or grams.

Standard Measurements

½ cup =	75w light bulb, woman's fist
1 cup =	baseball, man's fist
1 tsp =	ping pong ball, first joint of thumb
1 tbsp =	poker chip
2 tbsp (1 oz) =	golf ball, shot glass, index finger
1 oz. meat =	pack of dental floss, disposable lighter
3 oz meat =	deck of cards, palm of hand
3 oz fish =	checkbook, palm and fingers

How Much to Eat?

- Forget weighing and measuring.
- Approximate amounts are sufficient for healthy eating or even for dieting.
- Just use your eyes, or even just your imagination.
- Or you can use your hands as a guide. You always have them with you.

Use these handy visual guides for healthy portion control and for learning to eat "standard" serving sizes.

Cereals, bread, rice, and pasta – Eat 5-7 servings per day; one serving equals:

¾ cup flaked cereal =	baseball
½ cooked cereal =	75w light bulb, tennis ball
1 pancake or waffle =	CD
1 bagel =	can of tuna (3 oz.)
Slice of bread =	cassette tape, bar of soap
1 biscuit =	hockey puck
½ cup cooked rice =	light bulb, tennis ball

¾ cup cooked pasta =	man's fist
1 muffin, croissant =	baseball
3 cups popcorn =	3 baseballs, med. cantaloupe
½ cup crackers =	6 med crackers

Vegetables, cooked – Eat 5-7 servings per day; one serving equals:

1 cup salad greens, raw =	grapefruit, or two cupped hands
1 cup vegetables =	baseball, 6 asparagus spears, 7 or 8 baby carrots
½ cup starchy veggies =	cupcake wrapper, tennis ball, woman's fist
1 medium potato =	computer mouse
1 ear of corn =	length of yellow pencil
5 med olives (with pits) =	poker chip

Fruits – Eat 3-5 servings per day; one serving equals:

1 medium piece =	baseball
½ cup grapes, cherries, berries =	baseball, or 16
1 cup strawberries =	grapefruit, or 12
½ cup fruit, canned or raw =	light bulb, tennis ball, cupcake wrapper
length of a medium banana =	length of a yellow pencil
¼ cup dried fruit =	golf ball, large egg

Milk products and cheeses – Eat 1-3 servings per day; one serving equals:

1 cup (8 oz) milk, yogurt =	baseball
½ cup frozen yogurt, ice cream =	75w light bulb, tennis ball
1-½ oz hard cheese =	4 dice, nine-volt battery
1-½ oz grated cheese =	checkbook
1 tbsp (1 oz) butter or cr. cheese =	poker chip

Meat and fish, protein– Eat 1-2 servings per day; one serving equals:

3 oz. meat or tofu =	deck of cards
3 oz. fish =	checkbook
2 tbsp peanut butter, hummus =	golf ball, walnut
¼ cup nuts =	handful, 12 nuts

Fats – Eat 1-2 servings per day; one serving equals:

    1 tbsp olive or vegetable oil =   poker chip
    2 tbsp salad dressing, mayo =   ping pong ball

Prepared Food s – once per day is okay, less often is better

    1 cup canned soup, chili, stew =   baseball
    ½ cup boxed or frozen
       mac and cheese =   tennis ball
    1 hamburger with bun =   hockey puck
    4 oz. chips, nachos =   grapefruit
    1 restaurant sandwich =   8 stacked CD's
    1 burrito, sub sandwich =   6 inches long, thick as your hand
    1 oz chocolate =   pack of dental floss

26 Exchanging This Food For That

Experts agree that a balanced diet is one of the most important avenues to good health and vitality. What do they mean by "balanced diet?" Most would agree that they are referring to a balance between carbohydrates, proteins, and fats, from which one would also get a balance of vitamins, minerals, and phytonutrients. There is little consensus, however, on what exactly the balance between carbs, proteins, and fats should be. (see Chapter 4, "Carbs, Proteins, and Fats – How Much of Each?") Generally speaking, 40% of calories from carbs, 30% from proteins, and 30% from fats are considered reasonable proportions.

You are not likely to get a perfect balance in any one meal, but getting your carbs, proteins, and fats to even out over the course of a day is achievable. All that is needed is for you to become conscious of the nutrients in common foods and then look for a reasonable balance each time you eat,

- Close to a balance of nutrients is usually best.
- Even slight changes can make a big difference.
- Minor changes add up to big changes if you make it a habit
- Eating more fat relative to carbohydrates can mean you feel less hungry between meals.
- Eating more protein relative to carbohydrates may result in more energy during normal "slump" periods, like late afternoons.
- Fresh or frozen is usually better than prepared or boxed foods.
- Eating unprocessed foods can be easy once you learn a few basic cooking techniques.
- Some healthy alternatives are surprisingly easy and tasty.

Here is a list of foods showing estimates of the relative proportion of each nutrient and how exchanging one meal for another can make an enormous difference over the course of a day or a week. Try a few and see whether your energy and hunger patterns change.

(Note: Nutrient proportions below are relative to total calories and are educated guesstimates, based on average serving sizes.)

EAT THIS   **instead of**   **THIS**
(carbs / protein / fat)   (carbs / protein / fat)

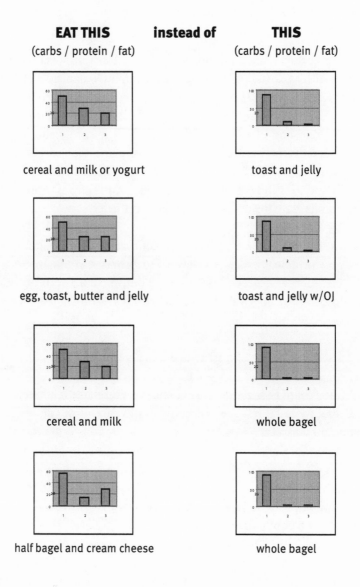

cereal and milk or yogurt   toast and jelly

egg, toast, butter and jelly   toast and jelly w/OJ

cereal and milk   whole bagel

half bagel and cream cheese   whole bagel

EAT THIS	**instead of**	**THIS**
(carbs / protein / fat)		(carbs / protein / fat)

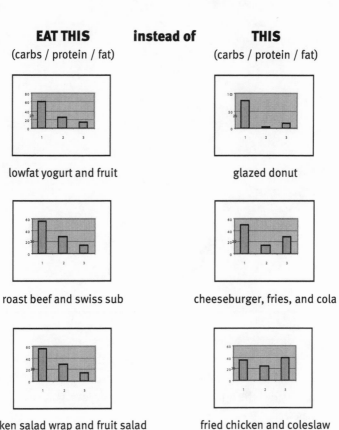

lowfat yogurt and fruit	glazed donut

roast beef and swiss sub	cheeseburger, fries, and cola

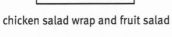

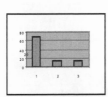

chicken salad wrap and fruit salad

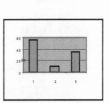

fried chicken and coleslaw

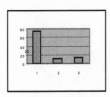

tortilla chips and guacamole

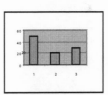

cheese and crackers

peanuts, pretzels, and beer

pizza and beer

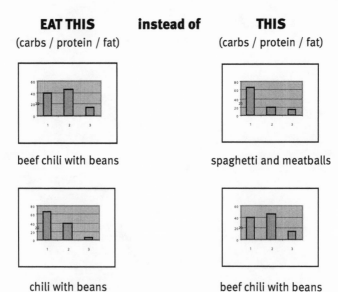

EAT THIS   **instead of**   **THIS**

(carbs / protein / fat)   (carbs / protein / fat)

beef chili with beans   spaghetti and meatballs

chili with beans   beef chili with beans

How about desserts? Most of us think desserts are bad for us because they are sweets. But mixing in a bit of fat with your sweets helps slow digestion and absorption, meaning you can avoid spikes in blood sugar and insulin. And if the added fat is nuts or chocolate, you've added some nutrition as well.

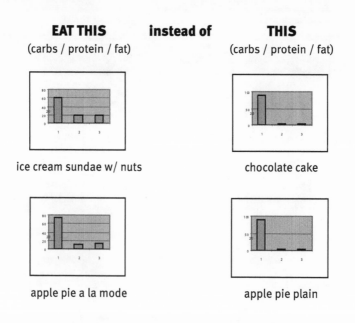

EAT THIS   **instead of**   **THIS**

(carbs / protein / fat)   (carbs / protein / fat)

ice cream sundae w/ nuts   chocolate cake

apple pie a la mode   apple pie plain

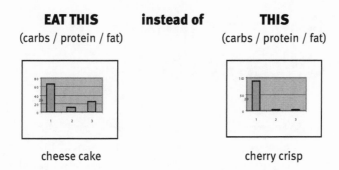

EAT THIS   **instead of**   **THIS**

(carbs / protein / fat)   (carbs / protein / fat)

cheese cake   cherry crisp

Maybe you are not so concerned about proportion of nutrients, but you are eager to minimize fat in your diet. Check out the following examples.

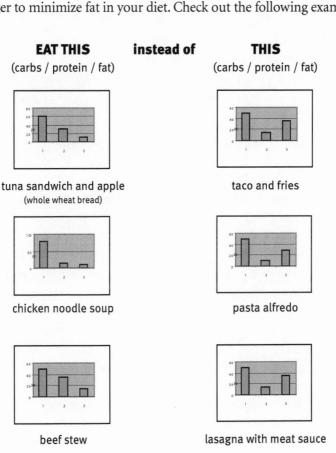

EAT THIS   **instead of**   **THIS**

(carbs / protein / fat)   (carbs / protein / fat)

tuna sandwich and apple   taco and fries
(whole wheat bread)

chicken noodle soup   pasta alfredo

beef stew   lasagna with meat sauce

27 Glycemic Index and Glycemic Load

The **Glycemic Index (GI)** is a measure of how fast carbohydrates are digested and absorbed into the bloodstream. Fast absorption = high glycemic index. Slow absorption = low glycemic index. How rapidly food is absorbed is affected by:

1. The type of carbohydrate in the food (simple or complex). See Chapter 3 – "What Foods are Made Of."
2. The presence of fiber (naturally, and in low – processed foods). See Chapter 12 - "Fiber in Your Food."
3. The presence of proteins and fats (lots of veggies have proteins and fats; fruits have none). Proteins and fats slow digestion and absorption.

   - A high glycemic index (rapid absorption) can cause spikes in blood sugar levels, especially dangerous for diabetics, but something most of us want to avoid.
   - So to avoid spikes in blood sugar, choose foods with a low Glycemic Index (GI).

The **Glycemic Load (GL)** is a measure of <u>both</u> the GI score and how much carbohydrate is in a typical serving. High carb = high glycemic load. Low carb = low glycemic load. Higher or lower scores are affected by:

1. The amount of water in the food (which affects volume).
2. How many calories per ounce are in the food (which reflects the presence of non-calorie fiber). See Chapter 24 – "Nutrient Density."
3. The amount of proteins and fats in the food relative to carbs (because proteins and fats slow the rate of absorption of carbohydrates through the small intestine into the bloodstream).
4. The size of a typical serving See Chapter 25 – "Serving Sizes and Portion Control."

Comparison of GI and GL Scores in Common Foods

- Foods with the most fiber, fat, and water have both low GI <u>and</u> low GL scores.
- On average, highly processed fruits and vegetables have higher GI scores than fresh, unprocessed fruits and vegetables.
- A high GI score means that the food is high in carbs and low in protein and fat. If you are watching your weight or carb intake, choose foods with a low GI score.

The table below with the **GI** and **GL** of a few common foods illustrates the relationship between **Glycemic Index** and **Glycemic Load**:

FOOD	GI	SEVING SIZE	NET CARBS	GL
Peanuts	14	4 oz (113g)	15	2
Bean sprouts	25	1 cup (104g)	4	1
Grapefruit	25	1/2 large (166g)	11	3
Pizza	30	2 slices (260g)	42	13
Lowfat yogurt	33	1 cup (245g)	47	16
Apples	38	1 medium (138g)	16	6
Spaghetti	42	1 cup (140g)	38	16
Carrots	47	1 large (72g)	5	2
Oranges	48	1 medium (131g)	12	6
Bananas	52	1 large (136g)	27	14
Potato chips	54	4 oz (114g)	55	30
Snickers bar	55	1 bar (113g)	64	35
Brown rice	55	1 cup 1951g)	42	23
Honey	55	1 Tbsp (21g)	17	9
Oatmeal	58	1 cup (234g)	21	12
Ice cream	61	1 cup (72g)	16	10
Macaroni & cheese	64	1 servng (166g)	47	30
Raisins	64	1 small box (43g)	32	20
White rice	64	1 cup (186g)	52	33
Sugar (sucrose)	68	1 Tbsp (12g)	12	8
White bread	70	1 slice (30g)	14	10
Watermelon	72	1 cup (154g)	11	8
Popcorn	72	2 cups (16g)	10	7
Baked potato	85	1 medium (173g)	33	28
Glucose	100	(50g)	50	50

1. Note that baked potatoes have a high **glycemic index**, but a comparably lower **glycemic load**; this is because they have a lot

of fiber in the skin and a fair amount of protein, which does not contribute to the **glycemic load**.

2. Similarly, watermelon has a high **glycemic index** but a low **glycemic load**, because watermelon has a lot of water in its flesh.

3. If you are trying to lose weight, select foods that have a low **glycemic load**.

4. If you wish to eat foods that satisfy your hunger longest, select foods with the lowest **glycemic index** because they take the longest to get into your bloodstream.

Look up individual glycemic index and glycemic load scores at:
www.health.harvard.edu
www.nutritiondata.com/topics/glycemic-index

28 Food is Everywhere!

Eating at Workplace, Sporting Events & Cocktail Parties

- How many times a day do you eat? Three meals a day? Three meals and three snacks?
- Eating is no longer an event, but an activity we typically enjoy while doing something else. Eating events now include:

  - mid-morning snacks
  - mid-afternoon nibbles in the break room
  - office gatherings to acknowledge achievements, birthdays
  - drinks after work
  - cocktail parties before a late dinner
  - quick fast food meals on our way to other obligations
  - store samples while shopping
  - tasting while cooking
  - sports events
  - picnics
  - potlucks
  - TV snacks

Research indicates that, on average, American adults eat six times a day. We have an opportunity to choose what to eat 48 times a week or more. No longer is a meal the typical unit of food consumption. A few bites at a time is more often the pattern for most of us. This has some advantages:

1. We don't experience hunger.
2. Energy levels are more stable throughout the day.
3. We have more choices of what to eat.

But some of those advantages can also be disadvantages:

1. We have become so accustomed to eating frequently that going a few hours without food seems abnormal.
2. We eat faster because all these extra food events take time out of our busy workday.

3. We eat more highly processed foods because they are convenient and quick.

Dieters report that keeping a food diary is an eye-opening experience. Most eating events are so entwined with other activities that we don't think of them primarily as eating. And they occur so often that dieters must carry pencil and paper everywhere.

- Colleagues take turns bringing doughnuts or bagels to work; this can turn into an every day activity. Even people who have eaten breakfast and are not hungry will be tempted by the sweets of doughnuts or the cream cheese accompanying bagels.

- Candy dishes appear on staff members' desks, especially following holidays like Hallowe'en and Valentine's Day—a way to share the bounty and, truth be told, get temptation out of the house. Soon candy dishes become a regular, anticipated part of the environment—a way to provide a moment of pleasure to passers-by.

- Some employers provide free drinks and snacks to workers—a way to keep them at their desks and energized, instead of walking to the vending machine or the diner or convenience store a block away for lunch or a snack.

- Coffee shops are ubiquitous – some coffee drinks can have as many calories as a modest meal. Drinking coffee throughout the day keeps us from getting hungry for "real" food.

- Fast food outlets are everywhere—rarely more than a few blocks from work or home. And the food there is often cheaper than eating fresh fruits and vegetables and home-cooked meals.

- "Let's go for a drink after work" becomes a tempting prospect as we slog through stressful, busy days with no time for interacting with colleagues, a chance to share "war stories" and develop friendships with people we see every day but know little about.

- It's not unusual for a shopper to encounter six or more food samples at the supermarket and specialty stores. So much food is frozen, bottled, packaged for quick preparation that food sellers must encourage buyers to sample their wares to tempt them to buy. Hungry shoppers are likely to think almost any prepared food tastes good.

- Shopping malls have centrally located food courts, wafting pungent aromas of hot, ready-to-eat, highly processed foods towards frenzied shoppers. It is too tempting for shoppers too busy and too tired to think about resisting begging kids and cooking something they won't like anyway.

How do we adapt to these changing patterns of eating? Should we? Are we ruining our health by eating so often? No one knows the answers to these questions, but a few common sense approaches come to mind. When presented with an eating opportunity:

1. Choose what and whether to eat deliberately and consciously.
2. If you are not hungry, decline—unless sheer pleasure is your goal. Then select what gives you the most pleasure.
3. If declining is taken as unfriendly, or even hostile, select a small portion and eat slowly.
4. Learn at least a little bit about various foods and your body's needs.
5. Cultivate an appreciation for what healthy foods do for you.
6. If you are hungry, choose what would give you the most pleasure. Your choice could be the one that tastes the best, satisfies your hunger the best, or is the most indulgent. If you have cultivated the above appreciations, the healthiest might be the most pleasurable and the most satisfying.

Bon appetit!

29 Using A Calorie Budget

If you struggle to control your weight, using a calorie budget might be helpful.

Eating means taking in calories. In a way, you are "spending" your calorie allowance as you eat throughout the day. You can use this metaphor to plan how you will allocate your calorie allowance in the same way you use a budget to plan how to allocate your paycheck.

You have just so much money to spend, and your body needs just so many calories to maintain a healthy weight. Just like building a budget for managing your finances, a calorie budget helps you manage what you eat in a planned, non-chaotic way. Like a financial budget, a calorie budget can be rigid and detailed or it can be casual and flexible. You get to decide.

The minimal requirements for a calorie budget are:

1. A sense of what your calorie needs are per day
2. A willingness to schedule and define eating events, even if you don't follow the schedule
3. Familiarity with the basics of nutrition requirements (this book can help with this one!)

Your calorie budget categories will reflect nutrition requirements, scheduled eating events, room for unexpected "expenditures," and unpredictable schedule changes. For this reason, I like to set up a budget for a week—long enough to allow averaging, approximations, and unexpected eating events, but short enough to not lose control of your eating patterns. Your calorie budget categories could include each regular meal and snack, unexpected events, predictable splurges, Saturday sports gatherings, monthly dinner parties, etc.

Steps for establishing your initial calorie budget (like any other budget, the basic structure will change as you gain experience over the time):

1. Determine your daily calorie requirement.
2. Decide on a basic daily eating pattern (e.g. breakfast, lunch,

dinner, 3 snacks; or 6 small meals per day; or a combination of those, or whatever), knowing that a planned eating pattern is just a guide for the week.

3. Decide on your goals for achieving optimal balance between carbohydrates, proteins, fats, empty calories, fiber and water. Experts disagree strongly on the appropriate proportion of each macronutrient. So you need to decide for yourself. For our example, we will keep it simple by using the rule of thirds:

1/3 CARBS	1/3 PROTEIN	1/3 FATS
1/3 unprocessed carbs	1/3 plant protein	1/3 saturated fat
1/3 processed carbs	1/3 meat/fish protein	1/3 monounsaturated fat
1/3 empty calories	1/3 dairy protein	1/3 polyunsaturated fat
(e.g. white sugar and flour in bread, pastries, desserts are all empty calories)		

4. Use a calendar and write in each food event for each day, however you want to eat. You can eat one meal a day if you want to, though I wouldn't recommend it. You'd have really tough extremes of being full and being hungry.

5. Take your total weekly calorie requirement, and allocate some calories to each event. For the most part, this will be the same every day. But you could allocate more calories to a weekend dinner, for example, than to the five weekday dinners.

6. Remember, this is all somewhat hypothetical, just like a financial budget. But it gives you a guide to go by and to deviate from. And if you do deviate, like going over your expense budget for Sunday breakfast, you know you have to take it from somewhere else.

A medium size woman might realistically decide that 1800 calories is a reasonable daily budget. Multiplying that by 7 gives a weekly calorie budget of 12,600 calories. You could allocate those calories as follows:

avg. breakfasts	300 cal	Or, you could decide: M-F	500 kcal/meal; 3 meals/day
avg. lunches	500 cal		100 per snack; 3 snacks/day
avg. dinners	700 cal	Weekends	800 kcal/meal; 2 meals/day
avg. snacks	100 cal		200 kcal/snack; 1 snack/day

This is how it would look on your calendar:

SUNDAY	MONDAY	TUESDAY	WEDNESDAY	THURSDAY	FRIDAY	SATURDAY
	Breakfast 300 kcal	Breakfast 300 kcal	Breakfast 300 kcal	Breakfast 300 kcal	Breakfast 300 kcal	Breakfast 300 kcal
Brunch 1050kcal	Mid-morning snack 100 kcal	Mid-morning snack 100 kcal	Mid-morning snack 100 kcal	Mid-morning snack 100 kcal	Mid-morning snack 100 kcal	Mid-morning snack 100 kcal
	Lunch 500 kcal	Lunch 500 kcal	Lunch 500 kcal	Lunch 500 kcal	Lunch 500 kcal	Lunch 500 kcal
Mid-afternoon snack 100 kcal	Mid-afternoon snack 100 kcal	Mid-afternoon snack 100 kcal	Mid-afternoon snack 100 kcal	Mid-afternoon snack 100 kcal	Mid-afternoon snack 100 kcal	
Dinner 600 kcal	Dinner 700 kcal	Dinner 700 kcal	Dinner 700 kcal	Dinner 700 kcal	Dinner 700 kcal	Dinner 900 kcal
Bedtime snack 100 kcal	Bedtime snack 100 kcal	Bedtime snack 100 kcal	Bedtime snack 100 kcal	Bedtime snack 100 kcal	Bedtime snack 100 kcal	

Of course, you'll say, that is ridiculously regimented. No one could or would want to follow such a plan. And you would be right. But having the plan allows you to figure out just what you ideally want to eat for any given meal or snack.

More importantly, when you deviate from the basic plan, you know that you have to add or subtract calories from somewhere else. Doing a budget for just a week at a time allows maximum flexibility. And best of all, it allows you to account for so-called "empty" calories—foods that have calories, but little or no nutrition.

Say you decide to have a dish of ice cream most evenings before bed. It's likely to be more than 100 calories. So you could systematically decide to move 100 of your dinner calories to your bedtime snack. But if you don't have a calorie budget, you would probably add the extra 100 calories of ice cream without taking the calories from anywhere.

Accounting for empty calories is like having an "entertainment" category in your household budget. If you didn't have one, every time you wanted to go out to the movies or dinner, you'd have to "borrow" the money from some other budget category. Same idea.

Once you get the hang of a calorie budget, you may choose to further refine your plan by figuring out how you will allocate your calories between carbs, proteins, and fats. You can do it right on your calendar, or you can just have it in mind when you are planning menus or choosing what to eat in restaurants. Once you get in the habit, it will become second nature. But if you never think about it and don't know how to do it, it won't become a new habit. Repetition is how new habits become familiar old habits.

Planned eating is happier eating. Enjoy!

30 Measurement Equivalents and Conversions

VOLUME		
ABBREVIATION	**MEASUREMENT**	**EQUIVALENTS**
Tsp	teaspoon	1 tsp = .17 fl oz 1 tsp = 4.93 ml
Tbsp	tablespoon	1 Tbsp = 1/2 fl oz 1 Tbsp = 3 tsp
fl oz	fluid ounce	1 fl oz = 29.573 ml
c	cup	1 c = 8 fl oz 1 c = 16 Tbsp
pt	pint	1 pt = 16 fl oz 1 pt = 2 c
qt	quart	1 qt = 4 c 1 qt = 2 pt 1 qt = .946 L
gal	gallon	1 gal = 4 qt 1 gal = 3.785 L
ml	milliliter	1 ml = 1/1000 L
L	liter	1 L = 1.057 qt

WEIGHT		
ABBREVIATION	**MEASUREMENT**	**EQUIVALENTS**
mcg	microgram	1 = 1/100,000 g
mg	milligram	1 mg = 1/1000 g
g	gram	1 g = .035 oz
kg	kilogram	1 kg = 2.2 lb
oz	ounce	1 oz = 28.35 g
lb	pound	1 lb = 16 oz 1 lb = .454 kg

31 Pesticides in Fresh Fruits and Vegetables

HIGHEST IN PESTICIDES	MEDIUM HIGH IN PESTICIDES	FAIRLY LOW BUT NOT PERFECT	LOWEST IN PESTICIDES
Buy organic if possible	Use caution and consider peeling before use, or using frozen or canned	Consider peeling before cooking. or using frozen or canned	Use after washing or peeling
Peaches	Spinach	Apple Sauce	Broccoli
Apples	Grapes	Raspberries	Orange Juice
Sweet Bell Peppers	Lettuce	Plums	Blueberries
Celery	Potatoes	Grapefruit	Papaya
Nectarines	Green Beans	Tangerine	Cabbage
Strawberries	Hot Peppers	Apple Juice	Bananas
Cherries	Cucumbers	Honeydew Melon	Kiwi
Carrots	Mushrooms	Tomatoes	Canned Tomatoes
Pears	Cantaloupe	Sweet Potatoes	Sweet Peas
Winter Squash (frozen)	Oranges	Watermelon	Asparagus
	Winter Squash (fresh)	Cauliflower	Mango
			Canned Pears
			Pineapple
			Sweet Corn
			Avocado
			Onions

Note: Foods were tested in a state they would be eaten by consumers—washed vigorously with water or peeled if the food is typically peeled, such as bananas.

- Pesticide use is at an all time high on commercial, non-organic agricultural production plants.
- For foods in the left-most column, try to buy only organic.
- Even the foods in the right two columns were not always found to be pesticide-free, but they were consistently low in pesticide residues and are your best bets for non-organic food.
- An environmental working group simulation showed that people can lower their pesticide exposure 90% by avoiding the most contaminated fruits and vegetables.
- Some pesticides are taken up internally by the plants and find

their way into the parts of the plant you eat; thus, the pesticides cannot be washed off.

- Other pesticides are designed to bind tightly to the surface of the fruit or vegetable so rain doesn't wash them off, which means you cannot easily wash them off either.
- Peeling does reduce exposure to surface-level pesticides for many of these foods, but you often lose valuable nutrients and roughage when you throw away the peel.
- The lists apply not only to fresh fruits and vegetables but often to the same items when they are in canned or frozen form, as well as to processed foods and restaurant meals that contain those particular fruits or vegetables.
- One large study found less contamination in processed food than fresh food; but you'll lose some of the valuable vitamins, enzymes, antioxidants, and other phytonutrients if you decide to avoid fresh food.

Sources: foodnews.org has a downloadable wallet size version of this list; whatsonmyfood.org has a search engine for you to find out exactly which pesticides are used on various types of fruits and vegetables, or you can search by pesticide.

32 Food Additives

Additives in processed foods are there for a number of reasons:
- Improve flavor or appearance (color, texture)
- Prevent spoilage and maintain freshness (increase shelf life)
- Control contamination
- Preserve and/or enhance nutritional value
- Minimize variations in flavor or texture

The Food and Drug Administration has approved many chemicals as food additives for several purposes:
- Coloring agents
- Natural and synthetic flavors
- Flavor enhancers
- Stabilizers
- Thickeners
- Sweeteners

Processed food manufacturers are required to list food additives (except color from natural sources) in their lists of ingredients. Fortified or enriched foods, particularly grain and dairy products usually have added vitamins and minerals. For example, milk has added Vitamins A and D, orange juice is fortified with Vitamin D and calcium, salt has extra iodine, and cereals often have added folate.

For centuries, ingredients have served useful functions in a variety of foods. Our ancestors used salt to preserve meats and fish, added herbs and spices to improve the flavor of foods, preserved fruit with sugar, and pickled cucumbers in a vinegar solution.

Today, processed food contains thousands of additives. The Food and Drug Administration (FDA) maintains a list of over 3000 additive ingredients in its data base "Everything Added to Food in the United States." All food additives are regulated by federal authorities and various international organizations to ensure that foods are safe to eat and are accurately labeled

Additives are thought to be harmless, except certain people may develop allergies to additives without knowing which ones. Limiting one's exposure to processed foods can avoid and/or alleviate this problem.

A list of all food additives approved by the FDA can be found at the following websites:

www.fds.gov/Food/FoodIngredientsPackaging/FoodAdditives/Food AdditiveListings/ucm091048.htm

www.fds.gov/Food/FoodIngredientsPackaging/ucm094211.htm#types

Sources: Hark, Lisa and Darwin, Deen. *Nutrition for Life.* DK. 2005;
           www.fda.gov

Types of Food Additives

TYPES OF INGREDIENTS	WHAT THEY DO	EXAMPLES OF USE	NAMES FOUND ON PRODUCT LABELS
Preservatives	Prevent food spoilage from bacteria, molds, fungi, or yeast (antimicrobials); slow or prevent changes in color, flavor, or texture and delay rancidity (antioxidants); maintain freshness	Fruit sauces and jellies, beverages, baked goods, cured meats, oils and margarines, cereals, dressings, snack foods, fruits and vegetables	Ascorbic acid, citric acid, sodium benzoate, calcium propionate, sodium erythorbate, sodium nitrate, calcium sorbate, potassium sorbate, BHA, BHT, EDTA, tocopherols (Vitamin E)
Sweeteners	Add sweetness with or without the extra calories	Beverages, baked goods, confections, table-top sugar, substitutes, many processed foods	Sucrose (sugars), glucose, fructose, sorbitol, mannitol, corn syrup, high fructose corn syrup, saccharin, aspartame, sucralose, acesulfame, potassium (acesulfame-K), neotame
Color Additives	Offset color loss due to exposure to light, air, temperature extremes, moisture and storage conditions, correct natural variations in color; enhance colors that occur naturally; provide color to colorless and "fun" foods	Many processed foods (candies, snack foods, margarine, cheese, soft drinks, jams/jellies, gelatins, puddings, & pie fillings)	FD&C Blue Nos. 1 & 2, FD&C Green No. 3, FD&C Red Nos. 3 & 40, FD&C Yellow Nos. 5 & 6, Orange B, Citrus Red No. 2, annato extract, beta-carotene, grape skin extract, cochineal extract or carmine, paprika oleoresin, caramel color, fruit & vegetable juices, saffron

TYPES OF INGREDIENTS	WHAT THEY DO	EXAMPLES OF USE	NAMES FOUND ON PRODUCT LABELS
Flavors and Spices	Add specific flavors (natural & synthetic)	Pudding & pie fillings, gelatin dessert mixes, cake mixes, salad dressings, candies, soft drinks, ice cream, BBQ sauce	Natural flavoring, artificial flavor, and spices
Flavor Enhancers	Enhance flavors already present in foods (without providing their own separate flavor)	Many processed foods	Monosodium glutamate (MSG), hydrolyzed soy protein, autolyzed yeast extract, disodium guanylate or inosinate
Fat Replacers (& components of formulations used to replace fats)	Provide expected texture and a creamy "mouth-feel" in reduced-fat foods	Baked goods, dressings, frozen desserts, confections, cakes & dessert mixes, dairy products	Olestra. cellulose gel, carrageenan, polydextrose, modified food starch, microparticulated egg white protein, guar gum, xanthan gum, whey protein concentrate
Nutrients	Replace vitamins & minerals lost in processing, (enrichment), adds nutrients that may be lacking in the diet (fortification)	Flour, breads, cereals, rice, macaroni, margarine, salt, milk, fruit beverages, energy bars, instant breakfast drinks	Thiamine hydrochloride, riboflavin,(Vitamin B2), niacin, niacinamide, folate or folic acid, beta-carotene, potassium iodide, iron or ferrous sulfate, alpha tocopherols, ascorbic acid, Vitamin D, amino acids (L-tryptopahn, L-lysine, L-luecine, L-methionine)
Emulsifiers	Allow smooth mixing of ingredients, prevents separation. Keeps emulsified products stable, reduces stickiness, controls crystalization, keeps ingredients dispersed and helps products dissolve more easily	Salad dressings, peanut butter, chocolate, margarine, frozen desserts	Soy lecithin, mono- and diglycerides, egg yolks, polysorbates, sorbitan, monostearate
Stabilizers & Thickeners, Binders, Texturizers	Produce uniform texture, improves "mouth-feel"	Frozen desserts, dairy products, cakes, pudding & gelatin mixes, dressings, jams & jellies, sauces	Gelatin, pectin, guar gum, carrageenan, xanthan gum, whey

TYPES OF INGREDIENTS	WHAT THEY DO	EXAMPLES OF USE	NAMES FOUND ON PRODUCT LABELS
pH Control Agents and acidulants	Control acidity and and alkalinity, prevents spoilage	Beverages, frozen desserts, chocolate, low acid canned foods, baking powder	Lacric acid, citric acid, ammonium hydroxide, sodium carbonate
Leavening Agents	Promote rising of baked goods	Breads and other baked goods	Baking soda, mono-calcium phosphate, calcium carbonate
Anti-caking agents	Keep powdered foods free-flowing, prevents moisture absorption	Salt, baking powder, confectioner's sugar	Calcium silicate, iron ammonium citrate, silicon dioxide
Humectants	Retain moisture	Shredded coconut, marshmallows, soft candies, confections	Glycerin, sorbitol
Yeast	Promote growth of yeast	Breads and other baked goods	Calcium sulphate, ammonium phosphate
Dough Strengtheners & conditioners	Produce more stable dough	Breads and other baked goods	Ammonium phosphate, azodicarbonamide, L-cysteine
Firming Agents	Maintain crispness and firmness	Processed fruits and vegetables	Calcium chloride, calcium lactate
Enzyme Preparations	Modify proteins, polysaccharides and fats	Cheese, dairy products, meat	Enzymes, lactase, papain, rennet, chymosin
Gases	Serve as a propellant aerate, or creates carbonation	Oil, cooking spray, whipped cream, carbonated beverages	Carbon dioxide, nitrous oxide

Source: www.fda.gov/Food/FoodIngredientsPackaging/ucm094211.htm#types

Some FDA-Approved Food Additives

CHEMICAL/PRODUCT NAME	PURPOSE
agar	thickener, texture
acesulfame potassium (acesulfame-k)	sweetener
alginate	thickener, texture
alpha tocopherols	nutrient
amino acids	nutrient
ammonium chloride	yeast food
ammonium hydroxide	acidity control
ammonium phosphate	yeast food
ammonium sulphate	dough conditioner
annatto extract	color additive

CHEMICAL/PRODUCT NAME	PURPOSE
ascorbic acid	preservative
ascorbic acid	nutrient
aspartame	sweetener
autolyzed yeast extract	flavor enhancer
azodicarbonamide	dough conditioner
baking powder	helps dough rise
baking soda	leavening agent
beta carotene	nutrient/color additive|
BHA	preservative
BHT	preservative
calcium carbonate	leavening agent
calcium chloride	firming agent
calcium lactate	firming agent
calcium propionate	preservative
calcium silicate	anti-caking agent
calcium sorbate	preservative
calcium sulfate	yeast food/nutrient
caramel color	color additive
carrageenan (Irish moss)	fat replacer/stabilizer
cellulose gel	fat replacer/texture
chymosin	enzyme
citric acid	preservative/acidity
Citrus Red No. 2	color additive
cochineal extract or carmine	color additive
corn syrup	sweetener
dextrin	thickener
disodium quanylate or inosinate	flavor enhancer
EDTA	preservative
egg white protein	fat replacer
egg yolks	emulsifier
FD&C Blue Nos. 1 and 2	color additive
FD&C Green No. 3	color additive
FD&C Red Nos. 3 and 40	color additive
FD&C Yellow Nos. 5 and 6	color additive
folate or folic acid	nutrient
fructose	sweetener
fruit and vegetable juices	color additive
gelatin	thickener, texture
glucose	sweetener
glycerin/glycerol	moisture retainer
grape skin extract	color additive
guar gum	fat replacer/thickener
high fructose corn syrup	sweetener
hydrolyzed soy protein	flavor enhancer
hydrolyzed vegetable protein	flavor enhancer
iron ammonium citrate	anti-caking agent

CHEMICAL/PRODUCT NAME	PURPOSE
iron or ferrous sulfate	nutrient
lactase	enzyme
lactic acid	acidity control
L-cysteine	dough conditioner
lecithin	enzyme
mannitol	sweetener
modified corn starch	fat replacer/prevents lumps
mono- and diglycerides	amulsifier
monocalcium phosphate	leavening agent
monosodium glutamate (MSG)	flavor enhancer
neotame	sweetener
niacin	nutrient
niacinamide	nutrient
Olestra	fat replacer
Orange B	color additive
papain	enzyme
paprika oleoresin	color additive
pectin	thicken, texture
phosphoric acid	acidity control
polydextrose	fat replacer
polysorbates	emulsifier
propylene iodide	nutrient
rennet	enzyme
riboflavin (Vitamin B2)	nutrient
saccarin	sweetener
silicon dioxide	anti-caking agent
sodium aluminum phosphate	firming agent
sodium benzoate	preservative
sodium carbonate	acidity control
sodium erythorbate	preservative
sodium hexametaphosphate	preservetive/moisture
sodium nitrate	preservative
sodium stearoyl-2-lactylate	preservative/emulsifier
sorbitan monostearate	emulsifier
sorbitol	sweetener/moisture retension
soy lecithin	emulsifier
sucralose (sugar)	sweetener
sulfur	preservative/prevents discoloration
tartrazine	color additive
thiamine hydrochloride	nutrient
tocopherols (Vitamin E)	preservative
Vitamin D	nutrient
whey	thickener, texture
whey protein concentrate	fat replacer
xanthan gum	fat replacer/emulsifier
sucrose/fructose	sweetener

33 Mercury in Fish

Lowest Mercury

Eat 2-3 servings a week (pregnant women and small children should not eat more than 12 ounces [2 servings] per week):

* Anchovies
* Catfish
* Clam
* Crab
* Crawfish
* Flounder
* Haddock

* Herring
* Mackerel
* Mullet
* Oyster
* Perch
* Pollock
* Salmon

* Sardines
* Scallop
* Shrimp
* Sole
* Squid
* Tilapia
* Trout
* Whitefish

Moderate Mercury

Eat six servings or fewer per month (pregnant women and small children should avoid these):

* Bass
* Carp
* Cod
* Halibut
* Lobster

* Mahi Mahi
* Monkfish
* Perch
* Snapper
* Tuna (canned chunk light)

High Mercury

Eat three servings or less per month (pregnant women and small children should avoid these):

* Bluefish
* Grouper
* Sea Bass
* Tuna (canned albacore, yellowfin)

Highest Mercury

Avoid eating (everyone):
* Marlin
* Orange Roughy
* Shark
* Swordfish
* Tilefish
* Tuna (ahi)

Sources: Food and Drug Administration (FDA). Mercury Levels in Commercial Fish and Shellfish
Centers for Disease Control. Public Health Statement for Mercury. Agency for Toxic
Substances and Disease Registry.

PART 3

Tips For Healthy Eating, Cooking, and Dieting

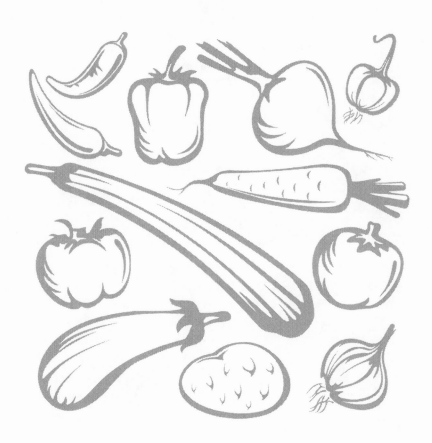

34 Tips For Healthy Eating, Cooking & Dieting

1. Add citrus or a splash of juice or infused tea to drinking water; sweeten with sweetener.
2. Add whole grains to diet gradually – pasta and bread come in whole grain versions that are made from half whole grain flour and half white flour.
3. Mix brown rice with white rice, or with wild rice to increase nutrition and fiber.
4. Avoid all sodas, especially diet sodas – empty calories and chemicals.
5. Eat fast food, junk food, any food without nutrition infrequently.
6. Balance your diet – eat 1/3 each of carbs, protein, fats (by calories, not grams); it's reasonable and easy to remember.
7. Before you indulge, ask yourself, is it worth it? Check your calorie budget. (See Chapter 29 – "Using a Calorie Budget.")
8. Black, green, and oolong teas are rich in polyphenols which boost insulin activity.
9. Brush your teeth after eating to discourage further eating.
10. Chew food thoroughly for better digestion and to slow your rate of eating.
11. Close down your kitchen after a certain hour.
12. Combine food that you don't like with items that you do; your taste preferences might change; butternut squash and kale make a great combination
13. Give yourself time to consciously choose satisfied over stuffed.
14. Consider that hunger is not an emergency; it is not life-threatening.
15. Consider whether you're really hungry when you are deciding to eat something.
16. Consume plenty of fiber to aid digestion and elimination.
17. Cultivate ways to be comfortable with the sensation of hunger – drink a little broth or watch the news before rather than during dinner.
18. Try to stop eating 3 hours before bed or 2 hours, at least. When we sleep, less food is converted to energy and more to fat.

19. Don't drink too much liquid with meals. It dilutes stomach acids for digestion, but drink lots between meals.
20. If you have a strong impulse to eat when you are really not hungry – out of stress, habit, emotional need or just because pleasurable food is offered, try cultivating an attitude of virtuous delay. Smug is okay sometimes.
21. Don't go into a meal starving – have a light snack before, preferably something with high water, low starch, like broth, or veggie appetizers.
22. Don't leave food in sight in your environment – candy dishes, fruit bowls, etc.
23. Don't let your waist size get larger than your inseam.
24. Don't skip meals – have a meal replacement shake if necessary.
25. Don't supersize at the fast food restaurant.
26. Don't use food to cure the blues, or if you do, do it consciously and deliberately; check to see if it really helps.
27. Don't waste calories on foods that don't add to your nutrition, unless the pleasure is worth it.
28. Eat all you want of non-starchy veggies: leafy greens, cucumbers, cabbage, cauliflower, and brocolli, etc.
29. Drink at least half an ounce of water or no-cal liquid per pound of body weight per day
30. Eat at the table – not at the computer or watching TV.
31. Eat before you get too hungry.
32. Eat a high protein breakfast; it's the most important meal of the day.
33. Eat foods in season; they will be more flavorful and satisfying.
34. Eat more raw fruits and vegetables – cooking kills healthy enzymes.
35. Eat negative calorie foods – celery and apples – that take more calories to digest than are consumed.
36. Try to eat protein, carbs and fat at every meal – balanced nutrients delay transit, slow digestion, increase satisfaction..
37. Eat slowly, let your stomach catch up to your hunger. It takes about 20 minutes for your body to register that it is full.
38. Save your treats for when you are away from home – dessert at restaurants, ice cream after a movie, etc.
39. Schedule a time in your week for treats – ice cream only on Saturdays, candy only at the movies, 2 cookies at bedtime.

40. Enjoy your food – consciously pay attention to how food looks and its smell, texture, and taste.
41. Establish eating habits and schedules that work for you; chaotic, unpredictable eating leads to unhealthy eating habits and overeating.
42. Consider exchanging your evening snack or meal for a larger morning meal. You'll probably sleep better, or, if hunger mars your sleep, try drinking a half cup of low-fat milk with a half cup of hot water.
43. Experiment with meal timing; some people do better with "grazing," eating 5 or 6 small meals a day; others do better eating full meals at approximately the same time most days; natural body rhythms vary considerably.
44. Get adequate nutrition – supplement with a natural multivitamin/mineral if you think you need it.
45. Limit simple carbs – high glycemic foods cause insulin spikes; treat them as a treat.
46. If hunger disturbs your sleep, eat 100-150 calories before bed and wait 20 minutes before trying to sleep.
47. If your sweet tooth calls, suck on hard candy–it prolongs sweet flavor and has few calories.
48. Instead of skipping a meal, drink a protein shake if necessary.
49. Keep evening snacks small – 150 calories or less.
50. Keep food in the kitchen – out of the bedroom, den or family room, desk, or car.
51. Keep healthy snacks available for appetizers when you get home, or for evening snacks – baby carrots, sticks of celery, radishes, jicama, sugar snap peas.
52. Learn enough about food and cooking to make good healthy choices, (use this book).
53. Limit white sugar, flour, bread, rice – the nutrition in overly processed foods has been stripped away.
54. Meditation can distract food cravings and reduce stress for some people.
55. Munch on a handful of nuts or seeds every day, especially walnuts which have lots of fiber and omega 3's. A mix of your favorite nuts and raisins or dried cranberries is a great snack.
56. Pack a lunch the night before to save time in the morning rush.
57. Reduce stress wherever you can – stress provokes the release of the hormone cortisol which facilitates fat storage.

58. Remove unhealthy snacks and desserts from your kitchen.

59. Make smoothies with yogurt and/or kefir and fresh or frozen fruits

60. Sometimes less variety is better than more; too many choices can be too stimulating; discover whether more or less variety works for you; this could even be different for different times of day or different circumstances; experiment and see how you feel.

61. Start the day by filling up as many containers as you need to equal 64 ounces of water; make sure they are all empty by bedtime.

62. Step outside during late day slumps for the same reason you use light in the morning; light can provide a quick pick-me-up in place of a snack.

63. Try drinking ½ cup of coffee or tea to counter the late afternoon slump, if you are not too sensitive to caffeine.

64. Take a power nap if you can.

65. Treat your other senses: watch TV, take a walk, get a massage, listen to music or talk radio or a book on tape; all will help distract you from cravings and appetites.

66. Try drinking ½ cup of coffee or other caffeine drink several times during the day, rather that one or two cups at a time; you can always drink half caf as a way of accomplishing the same thing.

67. Try packing lunch instead of eating out once a week, then twice, etc. – until you prefer it.

68. Try replacing restaurant meals with at home meals gradually: 1 per week, then 2, etc.

69. Try using light therapy during first hour you are awake (at least 12 minutes): take a walk; breakfast by a sunny window; sit on porch; crank up lights in the room you are in for the first ½ hour; use light therapy box. It may improve your mood and keep your daily rhythms in sync.

70. Try waiting an hour to eat even when you are hungry, to get used to the feeling – maybe you won't panic the next time you are really hungry.

71. Use a daily calorie budget (See Chapter 29 – "Using a Calorie Budget").

72. Use non-food alternatives to cope with stress: deep breathing, meditation, yoga, photo albums, music, write in journal, go for walk, work out, reading, watching TV, movie.

73. Monitor alcohol intake – a little can be good for you, but alcoholic

drinks are mostly empty calories.

74. When eating, try to focus on eating, not random thoughts

75. If you tend to rush in the morning, wind down in the evening by setting up breakfast things and packing lunch the night before.

76. Pick up pre-washed bags of salad greens and add baby carrots or grape tomatoes for a salad in minutes. Buy small packages of veggies such as baby carrots or celery sticks for quick snacks.

77. Use a microwave to quickly "zap" vegetables. White or sweet potatoes can be baked quickly this way.

78. Prepare more foods from fresh ingredients to lower sodium intake. Most sodium in our diets comes from packaged or processed foods.

79. Select vegetables high in potassium often, such as sweet potatoes, white beans, tomato products, beet greens, soybeans, lima beans, winter squash, spinach, lentils, kidney beans, and split peas. As much as limiting sodium intake, having a good ratio of sodium to potassium is important.

80. Eat frozen instead of canned vegetables for less salt. Buy canned vegetables labeled "no salt added." If you want to add a little salt, it will likely be less than the amount in the regular canned product.

81. Plan some meals around a vegetable main dish, such as a vegetable stir-fry, casserole or soup. Add small bits of meat as flavoring, if you wish.

82. Shred carrots or zucchini into meatloaf, casseroles, quick breads, and muffins. Include chopped vegetables in pasta sauce or lasagna.

83. Use pureed, cooked vegetables such as potatoes to thicken stews, soups and gravies. These add flavor, nutrients, and texture.

84. Grill vegetable kabobs as part of a barbecue meal. Try tomatoes, mushrooms, green peppers, and onions. Make fruit kabobs with pineapple, apples, melon, and grapes for dessert.

85. Buy fruits that are dried, frozen, and canned (in water or juice) as well as fresh, so that you always have a supply on hand.

86. Eat whole or cut-up fruit rather than drinking juice when you can. The extra fiber means fruit will be digested more slowly. If you do drink juice, make it 100% juice, rather than fruit drink or juice cocktail.

87. Select fruits high in potassium such as bananas, prunes and prune juice, dried peaches and apricots, cantaloupe, honeydew melon, and orange juice.

88. Keep a package of dried fruit in your desk or bag. Some fruits that are available dried include apricots, apples, pineapple, bananas, cherries, figs, dates, cranberries, blueberries, prunes (dried plums), and raisins (dried grapes). Better yet: mix dried fruit with a few nuts.
89. Offer kids fresh cut-up fruit (and a napkin) rather than fruit rope or fruit leather, which are high in sugar and low in real fruit.

Cooking Tips

1. Add minced garlic and salt and pepper to steamed veggies; the heat will cook the garlic just enough to infuse flavor into veggies.
2. Add pungent ingredients (balsamic vinegar, rough-ground pepper, savory herbs and spices, sweeteners, etc.) to enhance the flavor of foods.
3. Avoid fake fats like margarine – butter and mayonnaise taste better and have better fats.
4. Limit omega-6 oils – corn, sunflower, canola, soybean, peanut and safflower; use monounsaturated oils instead (olive oil, grapeseed oil). Most of us eat more than enough omega 6's.
5. Buy whole grains in bulk so you can get just what you will use in a week or two; whole grains have fat that can go rancid; alternatively, keep in refrigerator.
6. Canned beets are a versatile vegetable for salads or chopped and added to rice.
7. Choose oils with high heating tolerance for cooking – grapeseed and peanut oils.
8. Combine raw and cooked vegetables for a texture treat.
9. Combine salty and sweet in vegetable and meat dishes.
10. Cook with food in season and grown locally when possible.
11. Eat fruit and vegetables with every meal.
12. Buy organic produce when possible to avoid pesticides (See Chapter 31 – "Pesticides in Fresh Fruits and Vegetables").
13. Eggs are a perfect protein; use abundantly in cooking. There is no clear evidence that eggs raise cholesterol levels.
14. Frozen fruits, esp. mango or peach slices and berries, make a great evening snack; thaw in microwave.
15. Learn cooking basics even if you don't like to cook; it is often just as easy to prepare fresh food as heating processed food in microwave.

16. Make hot milk with half milk and half water.
17. Make smoothies with whey protein powder, low-fat milk, and one teaspoon frozen juice.
18. Mix nonfat or lowfat plain yogurt with sugar-free jelly or jam, instead of buying flavored yogurts.
19. Mix plain yogurt with thawed frozen fruits and a bit of sugarless sweetener.
20. Plain frozen strawberries, low-fat milk, and sweetener in the blender make a great shake; add other fruits, grains, yogurt or kefir, protein powder for a meal replacement drink; use either dairy, rice, almond, coconut, or soy milk.
21. Poach salmon in a little water and/or wine or cover and microwave for a quick healthy main course.
22. Put a couple of tablespoons of whole milk or half-and-half into cottage cheese; add sweetener and cinnamon—tastes a lot like rice pudding.
23. Replace frying with roasting, grilling, poaching, steaming.
24. Replace table salt with coarse sea salt in cooking.
25. If you do eat processed food products, try to choose those that have 5 ingredients or less.
26. Simmer broths to reduce volume and intensify flavor.
27. Simmer skinless chicken in a small amount of salted water until just done; freeze in serving sizes and use in recipes or chill and chop for chicken salad; nibbling on bones, cold or warm, can be a good meal or snack; chill broth until fat congeals, skim, and use broth for soup or to steam veggies, or mix with a boullion cube for a satisfying cold night drink.
28. Spice it up; use fragrant spices, chilis to stimulate taste buds and make low calorie food more satisfying (See Chapter 21 – "Spices and Herbs").
29. Sprinkle unsweetened shredded cocoanut and no-cal sweetener on frozen fruit for a sweet, low calorie dessert.
30. Sprinkle veggies with grated cheese, olive oil, chopped garlic, Tabasco, tomato or pesto sauce in enhance flavor.
31. Steam veggies in a bit of water with a pat of butter; cover, shake and drain; enough butter will coat the veggies for good flavor, but most will go down the drain.
32. Stock kitchen with healthy convenience foods (plain yogurt and

kefir, popcorn, frozen veggies and fruits, prewashed greens, serving size frozen brown rice, canned beans, tomatoes, whole grain wraps, precooked meats like sliced chicken or turkey).

33. Substitute a flavor-infused tea for soda; add sweetener if you prefer sweet tea.
34. Substitute apple sauce for oils when baking.
35. Substitute one whole egg and six egg whites for every 6 eggs in recipes.
36. Throw extra veggies into everything—sandwiches, eggs, casseroles, burgers, pizza, soups, frozen dinners, pasta, meat loaf. (Note: account for water when adding veggies to eggs and casseroles.)
37. Add chopped spinach to turkey burgers or meat loaf.
38. Mix shredded or chopped carrots, water chestnuts, and celery to tuna or chicken salad.
39. Double the amount of vegetables in soups.
40. Add peas, carrots, and/or diced or shredded zucchini to rice pilaf.
41. Toast nuts and seeds to accentuate flavor.
42. Trim visible fat from red meat and poultry, skin from chicken.
43. Use artificial sweetener on frozen fruit for a low calorie dessert.
44. Use meat as a side dish or as a condiment instead of main course, as in stir fried dishes.
45. Use fine mesh microwave cover in place of plastic wrap or paper towel (available in household goods stores).
46. Use precooked bacon; cut up one slice, sauté with veggies for tasty treat.
47. Use prewashed spinach; sauté in olive oil and a bit of garlic for a gorgeous veggie side dish.
48. Use tofu or beans as alternative sources of protein. (See Chapter 8 – "Getting Protein from Plants".)
49. Use unsweetened cocoa and sweetener for hot chocolate; drink it straight (like black coffee) or add hot milk or half-and-half to taste. Cocoa has a lot of antioxidants and is low calorie.
50. Use whey protein instead of soy protein powder if you are trying to avoid estrogen.
51. Whole fruit is better than juice – fiber moderates glycemic load
52. Make several meals on the weekend and heat up for dinner; don't do this if you hate leftovers.
53. Look for healthy convenience foods with low fat, calories, and so-

dium; use them for those times you are hungry and just too tired to cook even the quickest meal.

54. Anything ending in "ose" in the ingredient list is a pseudonym for sugar.

55. Try crushed, unsweetened whole-grain cereal as breading for baked chicken, fish, veal cutlets, or eggplant parmesan.

56. Use whole-grain bread or cracker crumbs in meatloaf.

57. Create a whole-grain pilaf with a mixture of barley, wild rice, brown rice, broth and spices. For a special touch, stir in toasted nuts or chopped dried fruit.

58. Experiment by substituting whole wheat or oat flour for up to half of the flour in pancake, waffle, muffin or other flour-based recipes.

59. Use whole grains in mixed dishes, such as barley in vegetable soup or stews and bulgur wheat in casserole or stir-fries.

60. For a change, try brown rice or whole-wheat pasta. Try brown rice stuffing in baked green peppers or tomatoes and whole-wheat macaroni in macaroni and cheese.

61. Use fresh fruit rather than chocolate or butterscotch on your ice cream; or make fruit sauce by simmering fruit with a bit of sweetener; or make chocolate sauce with unsweetened cocoa and sweetener

62. If you accidentally over-salt a recipe while it's still cooking, put in a peeled potato to help absorb some of the excess saltiness.

63. Cook whole-grain rice and pasta in large batches; divide into serving size pouches and freeze.

64. Add crushed pineapple to coleslaw or include mandarin oranges or grapes in a tossed salad.

65. For fresh fruit salads, mix apples, bananas, or pears with acidic fruits like oranges, pineapple, or lemon juice to keep them from turning brown.

66. Make a fruit smoothie by blending fat-free or low-fat milk or yogurt with fresh or frozen fruit. Try bananas, peaches, strawberries, or other berries. Add some protein powder for a nutritional boost.

Tips for Dieters

1. Drink an extra 16 ounces of water daily if you are actively dieting; water flushes waste products, helps digest food, helps you feel full, avoids overheating during exercise.

2. Avoid OTC diet aids; they provide short term help at best and can be dangerous if not used properly.
3. Avoid super strict diets; prohibitions set up cravings.
4. Be aware of eating triggers – stress, conflict, bad relationships, self worth.
5. Before beginning a diet, take steps to change habits of thought that will help you become ready for the change and to set realistic goals. Repetition helps build new habits.
6. Chart your weight loss weekly, but don't weigh daily; natural fluctuations in weight could cause discouragement.
7. Consult portion control visuals (See Chapter 25 – "Serving Sizes and Portion Control").
8. Don't compare yourself to anyone else.
9. Don't go cold turkey on favorite foods; establish modest goals using substitutes and plans.
10. Fill your subconscious mind with positive subliminal messages
11. Find a diet buddy for support and sharing and for exchanging commitments; it is easier to keep a promise to someone else than to yourself.
12. Get a decent scale.
13. Hypnosis / self hypnosis may work for you.
14. Identify emotional eating cues; make a list to help you realize what they are.
15. In a restaurant, request a box as soon as your meal arrives; put half of your food away before you begin eating.
16. Keep a journal of your food intake for a week or two, or even a few days, to get accurate and realistic information of what you are actually eating and to highlight places where substitutions may work for you.
17. Kick one vice at a time; don't try to give up smoking, caffeine, chocolate, or alcohol at the same time as food favorites.
18. Learn calorie counts by type of food and serving size, rather than trying to memorize calorie lists; approximation is a good strategy (see portion control tips).
19. Make a list of reasons that you want to lose weight
20. Make a list of rewards that you will give yourself when you lose a certain amount of weight.
21. Mix it up – your diet and exercise.

22. Order children's portions at restaurants.
23. Reward yourself with treats other than food – new clothes, a movie, a new book.
24. Serve food on individual plates rather than family style.
25. Set realistic diet and weight goals; unrealistic goals set you up for failure.
26. Split entrees and desserts at restaurants.
27. Split leftovers into single serving sizes before freezing.
28. Take before and after pictures (maybe some in between).
29. There is no bad food; pleasure is a legitimate reason for eating something; schedule treats, rather than trying to cut them out entirely.
30. Think about what you can add to your diet, rather than what you have to take away; use exchanges and substitutes (See Chapter 26 – "Exchanging This Food for That").
31. Use smaller dishes and utensils.
32. Visualize yourself being at your ideal weight / body shape.
33. Wait 20 minutes before taking seconds; it takes that long for your body to signal that you are full.
34. Serve snacks in bowls, rather than putting out a whole box of cookies or bag of chips.
35. Your stomach is about the size of your fist; eat portions accordingly.

PART 4

Staying Healthy

35 Digestion & Metabolism
How Bodies Process Food

Digestion, absorption, and metabolism is the process of breaking down food into its basic chemical constituents that your body can use to generate energy and build tissue.

1. Digestion takes place in the mouth and stomach: food is broken down in the mouth by chewing and in the stomach by churning.
2. Food particles are then made liquid by the addition of hydrocholoric acid from the stomach and enzymes and bile from the liver and pancreas.
3. Dissolved food moves into the small intestine, where all usable parts are absorbed into the bloodstream; indigestible residue moves on through the large intestine and is eliminated.

Parts of the Digestive System

Mouth (teeth, tongue, salivary glands)	Mechanical breakdown of food into smaller size chunks you can swallow without choking
Esophagus	Moistening and compacting food to facilitate swallowing
Stomach	Further mechanical breakdown by churning Release of enzymes, acid, and mucus to chemically break down food into absorbable liquid Begin protein and fat digestion
Liver Pancreas Gallbladder	Secrete pancreatic enzymes and bile into small intestine to complete final digestion of proteins into amino acids, fats into fatty acids and carbohydrates into absorbable glucose
Small intestine	Absorption of sugars, amino and fatty acids, vitamins, and minerals into bloodstream, where they are carried to the liver for distribution to cells, where they are metabolized (burned) for energy and used for cell and tissue repair
Large intestine	Absorption of water from indigestible residue to prepare for elimination
Rectum Anus	Elimination of indigestible residue

The absorption rate of food is determined in part by how quickly the body can convert its macronutrients into their simplest chemical constituents: simple carbohydrates (sugars) are converted the quickest, then complex carbohydrates, then proteins, then fats. Water soluble vitamins (all the B vitamins and Vitamin C) are absorbed more quickly than fat-soluble vitamins (A, D, E, K).

Fiber (indigestible residue) affects digestion by:
1. Delaying emptying of the stomach because food breakdown is slower
2. Slowing the passage of food through the small intestine
3. Blocking absorption of some nutrients
4. Indigestible residue (roughage) mechanically cleansing the walls of the large intestines

36 Keeping Cholesterol Levels Healthy

What is cholesterol?

- Cholesterol is a waxy, fat-like substance made by the liver from the fats we eat, and transported to the cells via the bloodstream.
- Your body needs some cholesterol to work properly. But if you have too much in your blood, it can stick to the walls of your arteries. This is called plaque.
- There are two main types of cholesterol: Low-Density Lipoproteins (LDL) and High Density Lipoproteins (HDL).

- **LDL cholesterol** is made up of particles of protein and fat that circulate in your blood delivering fats for cells to use for energy and body maintenance. Their low density makes them soft and sticky and likely to cling to artery walls and form deposits of plaque. Plaque deposits can become irritated and inflamed and burst open, allowing blood clots to enter the bloodstream and clog tiny arteries. When this happens, you are at risk for heart attack and stroke. Higher LDL cholesterol levels mean higher risk for cardiovascular disease.

- **HDL cholesterol** is known as "good" cholesterol because it helps prevent arteries from becoming clogged. As LDLs circulate through blood and cells delivering their fats, they become firmer and more dense—and convert to HDLs; these molecules are much less likely to stick to vessel walls.

- Plaque formation is why the **ratio of HDLs and LDLs** in your blood is the most important measurement in your Lipid Panel. Ideally, the ratio should be at least half as many HDLs as LDLs. Higher HDL cholesterol levels generally mean lower risk for disease.

The National Institutes of Health (NIH) recommends the following levels of cholesterol:

Total Cholesterol

Recommended level	<200 mg/dL*
Moderate health risk	200 – 239 mg/dL
High health risk	>240 mg/dL

*mg/dL = milligrams per deciliter

LDL cholesterol

Below 70 mg/dL	Ideal for people with many risk factors for cardiovascular disease (obesity, smoking, family history, high fat/calorie diet)
Below 100 mg/dL	Ideal for people with one or two risk factors for heart disease
100-129 mg/dL	Near ideal for people with no risk factors
130-159 mg/dL	Borderline high
160-189 mg/dL	High
190 mg/dL and above	Very high

HDL cholesterol

Good level	>60 mg/dL
Moderate health risk	50-59 mg/dL
Poor	<40 (men) and <50 (women) mg/dL

What are triglycerides?

- Triglycerides are a type of fat found in your blood.
- When you eat, your body converts any calories it doesn't need to use right away into triglycerides.
- The triglycerides are stored in your fat cells.
- Later, hormones release triglycerides for energy between meals.
- If you regularly eat more calories than you burn, particularly "easy" calories like carbohydrates and fats, the level of triglycerides in your blood will be high.

NIH-recommendation for healthy triglyceride levels:

Normal	< 150 mg/dL
Borderline high	150 to 199 mg/dL
High	200 to 499 mg/dL
Very high	500 mg/dL

So how do you improve your cholesterol and triglyceride numbers? (See also Chapter 10 – "All About Fats, p. xx)

1. **Don't overeat!** – Even if you avoid fats, eating excess calories of any kind, especially highly processed foods, raises cholesterol and triglycerides. Overeating occasionally is okay; it's excess calories every day that produce cholesterol test results that are unfavorable for health.

2. **Keep cholesterol-laden foods in your diet to a minimum** – fatty meat, shellfish, eggs, and full-fat dairy. Your body makes all the cholesterol you need, so you don't need to get it from food.

3. **Eat more plants than animals.** Plants have no cholesterol, even high fat plants like nuts and avocados. Plants have fiber which slows stomach emptying and absorbs some cholesterol in the small intestine. Plants do have natural compounds called sterols and stanols that mop up cholesterol in the intestines before it gets into the bloodstream.

4. **Exercise** – prolonged movement seems to improve cholesterol levels. It may be that fats are burned more efficiently during physical activity, or just that we use more of the calories we eat. In any case, any type of regular activity helps keep LDLs down and HDLs up.

Good Foods for Lowering Cholesterol and Triglycerides

(see Chapter 10 – "All About Fats" and Chapter 12 – "Fiber in Your Food").

1. *Oatmeal, oat bran and other high-fiber foods*

Oatmeal contains soluble fiber (6 g per serving), which reduces your low-density lipoprotein (LDL), the "bad" cholesterol. Other foods rich in soluble fiber are apples, barley, kidney beans, and prunes. An ideal diet contains 5-10 grams of soluble fiber daily.

2. Fish and other foods with omega-3 fatty acids

Eating fatty fish can be heart-healthy because of its high levels of omega-3 fatty acids, which can reduce your blood pressure and risk of developing blood clots. In people who have already had heart attacks, fish oil — or omega-3 fatty acids — may reduce the risk of sudden death.

Nutrition experts recommend eating at least two servings of fish a week. The highest levels of omega-3 fatty acids are in:

Mackerel	Albacore tuna
Lake trout	Salmon
Herring	Halibut
Sardines	

3. Walnuts, almonds and other nuts

Walnuts are the only nut with high amounts of omega 3's which can help reduce blood cholesterol. Rich in polyunsaturated fatty acids, nuts help keep blood vessels healthy.

According to the Food and Drug Administration, eating about a handful (1.5 ounces, or 42.5 grams) a day of most nuts, such as almonds, hazelnuts, peanuts, pecans, some pine nuts, pistachio nuts and walnuts, may reduce your risk of heart disease.

4. Olive oil

Olive oil is rich in antioxidants and monounsaturated fats that can lower your "bad" (LDL) cholesterol but leave your "good" (HDL) cholesterol untouched.

The Food and Drug Administration recommends using about 2 tablespoons (23 grams) of olive oil a day in place of other fats in your diet to get its heart-healthy benefits. To add olive oil to your diet, you can saute vegetables in it, add it to a marinade, or mix it with vinegar as a salad dressing (see Chapter 19 – "Cooking and Seasoning Oils").

5. Foods with added plant sterols or stanols

Foods are now available that have been fortified with sterols or stanols — substances found in plants that help block the absorption of cholesterol. Margarines, orange juice and yogurt drinks with added plant sterols can help reduce LDL cholesterol by more than 10 percent, but seem to have no affect on levels of triglycerides or HDLs.. The amount of daily plant sterols needed for results is at least 2 grams — which equals about two 8-ounce (237-milliliter) servings of plant sterol-fortified orange juice a day.

Sources: www.nih.gov; www.mayoclinic.com

37 BMI – Body Mass Index

- BMI is a measure of your weight relative to your height.
- Because BMI does not take into account degree of musculature, fat distribution or bone density, it is a very rough measure, only slightly more meaningful than traditional height/weight charts used by insurance companies.
- Much of the so-called obesity epidemic has been based on the distribution of BMIs in various age groups.

How to Calculate Your BMI:

$$BMI = \frac{weight\ (in\ pounds)}{height\ (in\ inches)^2} \times 703$$

According to the National Institutes of Health ...
"Underweight   =   BMI below 18.5
"Normal"   =   BMI 18.5 to 25
"Overweight"   =   BMI between 25 and 30
"Obese"   =   BMI over 30
"Morbidly obese" =   BMI over 40

These guidelines have serious limits. For example, using these guidelines, an athlete or body builder with lots of muscle (which weighs more than fat) could easily have a BMI over 30 and be considered obese; and a model with "normal" blood chemistry and low body fat could have a BMI under 18.5 and feel exceptionally good, but be labeled underweight.

To calculate disease risk relative to obesity or BMI, one must also consider:
- fitness level – including stamina, resting heart rate, etc.
- body fat percentage – how much of one's body mass is fat
- body fat distribution – whether fat is subcutaneous (just below the skin), or visceral (surrounding internal organs)
- bone density – can vary considerably by body type and amount of exercise a person gets

38 Hormones

Hormones are chemicals secreted in tiny amounts by a variety of different cells, organs, and glands in response to changes in physiological status. They work 24/7. They regulate every process in the body.

- There are hundreds, if not thousands, of different hormones.
- Hormones carry chemical messages between brain, organs, glands, muscles, and cells.
- Hormones influence, and are influenced by, other hormones, as well as other body chemicals.
- Hormone interactions are complicated, following multiple physiological pathways.
- Hormones function best when levels are in equilibrium; optimal levels change as we age.
- Hormone secretions are inhibited, enhanced, or blocked by changes in body status:

  - Temperature
  - Stress
  - Eating behavior
  - Illness
  - Obesity
  - Other hormones
  - Presence of toxins (pesticides, drugs, etc.)
  - Disruptions in normal rhythms

Major hormones are divided into four main categories:
1. **Sex** (reproductive) hormones: estrogen, testosterone, progesterone
2. **Metabolic** (energy) hormones: thyroid, insulin, growth hormone, leptin, ghrelin
3. **Regulatory** (rhythm) hormones: aldosterone, melatonin, parathyroid
4. **Stress** (emotional) hormones: cortisol, epinephrine, norepinephrine

The brain, particularly the hypothalamus, is the master regulator of hormone secretions. The brain sends chemical messengers—neurotransmitters—via the nervous system to glands, organs, and cells telling them to secrete hormones. Therefore, neurotransmitter levels in the brain also influence hormone levels and equilibrium.

Metabolic hormones regulate:
1. Hunger/appetite
2. Food digestion
3. Nutrient absorption
4. Metabolism rate
5. Nutrient transport into cells
6. Satiety – the feeling of fullness

Metabolic hormones are secreted by:
1. Brain
2. Pancreas
3. Thyroid
4. Stomach and intestine linings
5. White adipose tissue (body fat)

Hormones affect eating behavior by:
1. Stimulating or suppressing appetite
2. Delaying or facilitating stomach emptying
3. Influencing whether dietary fat is used for fuel or stored as fat
4. Influencing whether stored fat is used for fuel
5. Affecting metabolic rates over time
6. Facilitating metabolism of food for energy
7. Signaling satiety, the feeling of being satisfied

Hormones Related to Eating, Weight Control, and Metabolism

HORMONE	FUNCTION
gastrin	Released by cells in the stomach and duodenum; stimulates the stomach to secrete gastric juices
somatostatin	Secreted by cells in the stomach; inhibits the release of gastrin and hydrochloric acid; in the duodenum inhibits the release of secretin and cholecystokinin; in the pancreas it inhibits the release of glucagon.

HORMONE	FUNCTION
Secretin	Secreted by cells in the duodenum when they are exposed to the acidic contents of the emptying stomach; stimulates the pancreas to secrete bicarbonate into the pancreatic fluid (thus neutralizing the acidity of the intestinal contents).
Cholecystokinin (CCK)	Secreted by cells in the duodenum and jejunum when they are exposed to food; acts on the gall bladder stimulating it to contract and force its contents of bile into the intestine; stimulates the release of pancreatic digestive enzymes; gives a satiety signal to the brain.
Glucagon-like peptide-1 (GLP-1) and glucose-dependent insulinotropic polypeptide (GLP)	Called incretins; enhance the ability of glucose to stimulate insulin secretion by the pancreas; stimulate the ability of the tissues (e.g., liver and muscle) to take up glucose from the blood; slows the emptying of the stomach; suppresses glucagon secretion; suppresses appetite.
Ghrelin	Secreted by endocrine cells in the stomach, especially when one is hungry; acts on the hypothalamus to stimulate feeding, counteracting the inhibition of feeding by leptin and PYY3-36.
Neuropeptide Y (NPY)	Secreted by neurons in the hypothalamus; a potent feeding stimulant; causes increased storage of ingested food and induces a calming effect in laboratory animals exposed to stressful situations.
Adiponectin	Secreted by visceral fat(fat surrounding organs); discourages body from using stored fat as fuel; stimulates appetite; part of feedback system to assure a stable supply of glucose to the brain.
Peptide YY3-36 (PYY3-36)	Released by cells in the intestine after meals; a potent feeding inhibitor; acts on the hypothalamus to suppress appetite, the pancreas to increase its exocrine secretion of digestive juices, and the gall bladder to stimulate the release of bile. Level of PYY3-36 is directly related to amount of protein eaten.
Leptin	Secreted by the fat cells, is part of a feedback system that informs the brain of the amount of bodyfat. Low levels of leptin signal the brain that the organism is starving.
Insulin	Secreted by pancreas; facilitates transport of glucose into cells; chronically high levels of insulin, due to insulin resistance, keeps appetite stimulated.

HORMONE	FUNCTION
Thyroxine	Secreted by thyroid gland; regulates basal metabolism rate, which increases when heat is required; excess dietary calories results in excess heat; imbalance of thyroxine can cause increased or decreased appetite.
Cortisol	Secreted by adrenal glands in response to stress and according to your natural circadian rhythm; increases appetite as body prepares for fight or flight.
Estrogen	Secreted by ovaries; decline in estrogen concentration results in gain in the body weight because when estrogen levels fall, the body tries to get estrogen from other sources. Fat cells produce estrogen, so the body stores extra fat in order to raise its estrogen level.

For detailed information about the endocrine system, hormone balance, obesity and other nutrition-related illnesses, see:

Greene, Robert A. and Leah Feldon. *Perfect Balance.* Clarkson/Potter. 2005. An excellent summary of how hormones function, and how to achieve optimal hormone balance through healthy diet and lifestyle. Good summary of common illness associated with hormone imbalance.

Isaacs, Scott, with Todd Leopold. *Hormonal Balance.* Bull Publishing. 2002. Explains the interaction of hormones, weight, and metabolism and provides menu recommendations for healthy eating.

Talbott, Shawn. *The Cortisol Connection: Why stress makes you fat and ruins your health.* Hunter House. 2002
A good summary of hormones that affect weight. Explains the connection between stress hormones, appetite, and eating behavior.

39 Nutritional Supplements
Why People Take Them and What They Do

Health food stores, vitamin stores, gyms, and countless catalogs and websites sell a dizzying variety of supplements in addition to vitamins and minerals. Now these supplements, with unfamiliar, scientific-sounding names, are showing up in grocery stores and discount stores. Why are they so popular, why are people taking them, and what do they do?

There are five main types of supplements, besides vitamins and minerals, as well as every combination of nutritional booster you can imagine:

1. amino acids
2. essential fatty acids
3. phytonutrients (phytochemicals of various kinds)
4. antioxidants
5. hormones

Here is just a sampling of the most common supplements you can find in your neighborhood health food or vitamin and mineral store:

Amino Acids

- the body needs 22 different amino acids to make the 50,000+ proteins in our bodies
- two categories: (non essential does not mean unnecessary)
  - essential amino acids – the body can't manufacture them; they must come from our diets and/or supplements
  - nonessential – the body makes them from essential amino acids
- supplemental amino acids are often used by athletes and body builders because they are believed to promote formation of muscle tissue

ESSENTIAL AMINO ACIDS	RDA (mg per kg of body weight)	RDA for 150 lb adult (in mg)	INFANT RDA (mg per kg of body weight)	CHILD RDA (mg per kg of body weight)
Histidine*	5-7	900	33	16.2
Isoleucine	12	900	80	28
Leucine	16	1200	128	42
Lysine	12	1050	97	44
Methionine	12	900	ND	ND
Phenylalanine	14**	1000**	ND	ND
Threonine	8	600	63	28
Tryptophan	3	300	19	4
Valine	14	900	89	25

* Essential for children; non-essential fr adults
** Not officially established. These are the amounts that are commonly used.
ND = Not officially determined.
Note: If you take supplements for essential amino acids, use free-form versions, which are absorbed more readily than amino acids in combination.

Non-essential Amino Acids (the body makes these)

Arginine	Glutamic acid
Alanine	Glutamine
Asparagine	Glycine
Aspartic acid	Proline
Carnitine	Serine
Citrulline	Taurine
Cysteine	Tyrosine

Amino Acid Supplements

AMINO ACIDS	BEST FOOD SOURCES	PURPOSE	SUPPLEMENTS AVAILABLE
Arginine	Chocolate, nuts, seeds, beer, oats, peanuts, soybeans	Stimulates immune system Heals wounds Slows cancer progression Builds creatine, with methionine and glycine	Arginine Methinine Glycine
Carnitine	Made by the body from methionine and lysine	Helps cells produce energy May help angina Helps CFS (chronic fatigue syndrome) Lowers triglycerides and LDL	Acetyl-L-Carnitine (ALC)

AMINO ACIDS	BEST FOOD SOURCES	PURPOSE	SUPPLEMENTS AVAILABLE
Creatine	Made by liver and kidneys from methionine and glycine Meat and milk	Helps build muscle Helps body replenish ATP (adenosine triphosphate)	Creatine 20-25 g a day to start; then 2-5 g a day
Cystine	Eggs, meat, dairy products, whole grains	With glutathione, clears toxins from body	N-acetyl-L-cysteine (NAC)
Glutamine	Abundant in animal and plant protein	Keeps digestive system, esp small intestine, healthy	Glutamine
Lysine	Fish, lean meats, chicken, soy products, milk, cheese, beans	With arginine, used to treat herpes viruses Interferes with insulin production	Lysine 2000-3000 mg (avoid if you have diabetes)
Methionine	Eggs, fish, milk, and meat	Makes cysteine Keeps cholesterol low Antioxidant	L-methionine 500 mg
Taurine	Made by the body from methionine and cysteine Meat and milk	Helps heart rhythms Antioxidant	Taurine-up to 300 mg (may depress CNS-central nervous system)
Tryptophan	Turkey, eggs Peanuts Avocados, oranges, bananas, cottage cheese, fish, lean meat	Used by the body to make serotonin and melatonin Sleep aid	Tryptophan, 5-HTP-300-400 mg
Phenylalanine & Tyrosine	Nuts and seeds, cheese, lima beans, avocados, bananas	Used for making epinephrine, norepinephrine & dopamine May help depression	Phenylalanine Tyrosine (avoid both if you have high blood pressure or are taking MAO inhibitors)
Tyramine	Aged cheeses, avocados Bananas, beer, beans, chocolate, nuts	Can trigger migraines Raises blood pressure	Tyramine (avoid if you get migraines)

Fatty Acids

Two fatty acids are called essential because you must get them from food; your body can't make them:
- Linolenic acid – also known as **Omega-3**
- Linoleic acid – also known as **Omega-6**

These two fatty acids make all the other fats, which you also get from your food.

A healthy balance of omega-6 and omega-3 fatty acids is essential because:
- They both make prostaglandins, hormone-like substances needed to regulate many body processes.
- Some prostaglandins regulate blood pressure, heart rhythms, kidneys, and digestion. Others produce inflammation, pain, and swelling.
- Although inflammation and swelling are necessary for healing injury, an excess of prostaglandins that produce these symptoms can cause chronic excessive inflammation.

Omega-6 fatty acids (linoleic acid) are common in foods; it is easy to get enough or even too much. There are three types:
1. Gamma-linoleic acid (GLA) – corn, safflower, sunflower, and soybean oils; makes non-inflammatory prostaglandins
2. Arachidonic acid –found in meat and milk; makes prostaglandins that cause inflammation and swelling
3. Dihomo-linoleic acid

Omega-3's (linolenic acid) are less common; it is important to make sure you get enough. There are three types:
1. Alpha linolenic acid – (ALA) found predominantly in plant foods, especially flaxseed.
2. Eicosapaentenoic acid (EPA) – found in fish oil; also made by the body from ALA.
3. Docosahexanoic acid (DHA) – found in fish oil; also made by the body from ALA.

EPA and DHA make non-inflammatory prostaglandins, helpful in a variety of body processes.

Fatty Acid Supplements: EPA and DHA in fish oil supplements

They work together to lower triglycerides which can lower chronic inflammation, thereby lowering the risk of heart and cardiovascular diseases, as well as arthritis symptoms like stiffness, joint tenderness and pain.

(See Chapter 10 – "All About Fats" for more information on essential fatty acids.)

Antioxidants

Antioxidants are substances in the body that neutralize free radicals—molecules with an extra atom of oxygen left over from metabolism. Free radicals are implicated in heart disease, diabetes, high blood pressure, and cataracts. Glutathione is believed to be the most powerful antioxidant, with Alpha Lipoic Acid a close second. Almost equally powerful in mopping up those pesky oxygen atoms are phytochemicals called flavonoids and carotenoids, listed below.

Glutathione (GSH) – Considered the most effective of antioxidants, glutathione is a tripeptide made by your body from three amino acids – cysteine, glycine, and glutamic acid, in the presence of selenium. You need all of these substances to make enough glutathione.

Antioxidant Supplements

NAME	BEST FOOD SOURCES	PURPOSE	RDA	SUPPLEMENTS
Glutathione	Broccoli, cabbage brussels sprouts, kale, cauliflower, parsley. Note: Glutathione is destroyed by cooking; eat some veggies & fruits raw	Counteracting free radicals and toxins that get into your body from food, air, etc.	100 mg	Glutamine 1000-5000 mg N-acetyl cysteine (NAC) Vitamin B2, & C, and Selenium Alpha-Lipoic Acid 200 mg
Alpha-Lipoic Acid	Made by the body	Helps recycle glutathione; helps mitochondria turn glucose into energy Combats diabetic neuropathy	200 mg	Alpha-Lipoic Acid 200 mg; up to 1800 mg per day if diabetic

Flavonoids

NAME	BEST FOOD SOURCES	PURPOSE	RDA	SUPPLEMENTS
Quercetin	Broccoli, red onions, shallots, apples, black tea, grapefruit, red wine	Combats free radicals Reduces inflammation and swelling Kills viruses, blocks allergies	ND	200-400 mg 3 tmes a day
Catechins	Green & black tea, red wine	Helps make platelets less sticky Anti-bacterial Cancer prevention	ND	Green tea extracts with at least 30% catechins
Alliin Allyic sulfide	Garlic and onion	Antioxidant, esp. capturing peroxyl free radicals Combats sticky platelets Lowers cholesterol Lowers blood pressure	1-3 fresh cloves	Dried garlic-300mg Aged garlic-7 g Note: aged garlic does not contain alliin, but does have the other antioxidant compounds
Anthocyanins	Blueberries, blue grapes, plums, red wine	Protects against retinal eye problems like macular degeneration and night blindness	ND	Bilberry supplements containing 25% bilberry 40-240 mg
Resveratrol	Red wine, purple grape juice	Lowers cholesterol Prevents blood clots Blocks Cox-2, which causes colon cancer	1-2 glasses a day or 1.5-3 cups of grape juice	Resveratrol-500 mg
Pro-Anthocyanins	Cranberries, red wine, purple grape juice, blueberries	Traps hydroxyl free radicals Helps poor circulation Protects against infections, esp UTI	ND	OPCs-50-300 mg
Capsaicin	Hot peppers	Blocks pain temporarily	ND	
Rutin	Citrus fruits, red wine, berries, buckwheat	Helps poor circulation	ND	Rutin- 2000-6000 mg
Hesperidan	Citrus fruits		ND	

NAME	BEST FOOD SOURCES	PURPOSE	RDA	SUPPLEMENTS
Naringin	Citrus fruits, esp. grapefruit	Helps poor circulation	ND	
Gingko biloba	From ginko biloba tree	Improves memory Helps blood flow to brain Prevents or reduces tinnitus	ND	Ginko biloba extract with 24% flavone glycosides & 6% terpene lactones – at least 40 mg up to 240 mg

Carotenoids (Carotenes and Xanthophylls)

NAME	BEST FOOD SOURCES	PURPOSE	RDA	SUPPLEMENTS
Alpha carotene	Carrots, sweet potatoes, squash, leafy greens, broccoli, apricots, cantaloupe	Removes singlet oxygen free radicals; stronger free radical than beta carotene Anticarcinogenic	ND	
Beta crypto-xanthin	Oranges, mangoes, papayas, cantaloupe	Removes singlet oxygen free radicals	ND	
Lycopene	Tomatoes, watermelon, pink grapefruit	Protects against cancer, esp. prostate, colon, lung Protects against cataracts and age-related macular degeneration and cataracts	6.5 mg	Lycopene supplements
Lutein	Green leafy vegs, esp. broccoli, kale and spinach; egg yolks	Especially protective against age-related macular degeneration	15-30 mg	Lutein supplement
Zeaxanthin	Green leafy vegs, esp. kale and spinach Egg yolks	Especially protective against age-related macular degeneration and cataracts	ND	Not available in supplements
Capsanthin	Green leafy vegs, esp kale and spinach, and red peppers	Protects eyes against cataracts	ND	Capsanthin supplements Cayenne capsules

Note: Carotenoids are fat soluble, so eat with a bit of fat, like olive oil.

Enzyme and Hormone Supplements

NAME	BEST FOOD SOURCES	PURPOSE	RDA	SUPPLEMENTS
Coenzyme Q10 (ubiquinone)	Oily fish Organ meats Soybean & canola oils Wheat germ Tofu	Helps mitochondria metabolize glucose Combats heart disease Makes platelets less sticky Lowers blood pressure	100-300 mg	Coenzyme Q10 oil based gel-caps 100-300 mg day, esp. if you have heart disease or diabetes, or are taking statins for cholesterol
Melatonin	Made by the pineal gland, using tryptophan Turkey Eggs	Helps restore normal sleep rythms Helps with jet lag	Made by the body	Melatonin-100-400 mcg 2-4 hours before bedtime (up to 3 mg)
Isoflavones (phytoestrogen, genistein, diadzein, ipriflavone)	Foods made with soybeans–tofu, soy milk, tempeh	Relieves menopause symptoms by blocking estrogen receptors Prevents osteoporosis and some cancers	20-50 mg	Isoflavone supplements –200 mg Ipriflavone supplements –600 mg Also calcium, boron, and Vitamin D
DHEA (dehydroepian-drosterone)	Made by adrenal glands No foods contain DHEA	Prevents osteoporosis Protects from side effects of steroids Relieves depression Used to treat auto-immune diseases like lupus and CFS*	ND	DHEA

Note: Two other hormones, Pregnenolone, and Human Growth Hormone, do not occur in food and are made in sufficient quantity by the body. However, they are believed to increase athletic performance, and their precursors are available as supplements in health food stores.
* Chronic Fatigue Syndrome

Pain Relief Supplements – Natural Compounds and Herbs

NAME	PURPOSE	SUPPLEMENTS
Glucosamine	Provides raw materials to rebuild damaged cartilage Reduces swelling	Glucosamine sulfate 500 mg 2 or 3 times per day Also Vitamin C and manganese

NAME	PURPOSE	SUPPLEMENTS
Chondroitin	Provides raw materials to rebuild damaged cartilage, though difficult to absorb	Chondroitin Sold in combination with glucosamine
SAMe (S-adenosyl-methionine)	Reduces swelling Also may help depression	SAMe – 1600 mg per day
EPA & DHA (omega 3's)	Reduces inflammation of rheumatoid arthritis	Fish oils – 6 g per day
GLA (Gamma-linoleic acid; omega 6)	May help pain of rheumatoid arthritis	Evening Primrose or Borage oil 1.4 – 2.8 g per day
DMSO (dimethyl sulfoxide)	Used to treat interstitial cystitis Used to treat sprains and aching joints	DMSO
MSM (methyl sulfonyl methane)	Relieves pain of arthritis, sore muscles, allergies	MSM – 3 g per day Sold combined w/ glucosamine
CMO (cetyl myristoleate)	Relieves pain of rheumatoid arthritis	CMO – 100 mg 2 – 4 times per day
Devil's Claw	Relieves pain	Devil's Claw (harpagophytum procumbens) 3% iridoid glycosides; 750 mg 3 times per day
Boswellia	May help relieve inflammation and protect cartilage	Boswellic Acids – 37.5% 400 mg 3 times per day
Bromelain	Enzyme found in pineapple; anti-inflammatory	Bromelain 1200 – 1800 mg per day
Turmeric	Powerful anti-inflammatory agent used to treat rheumatoid arthritis	Curcumin 400 mg 3 times per day

Miscellaneous Supplements

NAME	BEST FOOD SOURCES	PURPOSE	SUPPLEMENTS
Turmeric	Mustard	Migraine pain relief	Turmeric
PS Phospha-tidylserine	No food contains PS	Protects cell membranes in the brain Improves memory Help for Alzheimer's disease	PS – 100 mg 3 times per day

NAME	BEST FOOD SOURCES	PURPOSE	SUPPLEMENTS
Huperzine A	Made from club moss	Treatment for Alzheimer's disease	Huperzine A
Vinpocetine	Made from periwinkle plant	Treatment for Alzheimer's disease	Vinpocetine
Acetyl-L Carnitine (ALC)	Made by the body	Needed to produce neurotransmitter acetylcholine, needed for cognition & memory	ALC – 750 mg 2 or 3 times per day
DHA and AA	Oily fish Also made by the body from ALA – alpha linolenic acid	Improves blood lipids levels Prevents or delays dementia in the elderly	Fish oil capsules and liquids

40 Nutritional Healing

Illnesses That May Benefit from Vitamin & Mineral Supplements

ILLNESS	HELPFUL VITAMINS Look for this minimum in multivitamin	HELPFUL MINERALS Look for this minimum in multimineral	HELPFUL FOODS	SUPPLEMENTS	AVOID OR REDUCE
Acne	Vitamin C 1000 mg 2x per day Niacin (B3) 100 mg x 30 days	Zinc 15 mg Sulphur	Eggs Onions Garlic Fruits and vegetables		Sugar Cigarettes Fried food High fat food
Alcoholism	Vitamin B1, B2, B3, & B6 Vitamin C 1000 mg 2x per day	Calcium 500 mg Magnesium 300 mg	Fruits and vegetables	Glutamine powder, 5 g	
Anemia	Cobalamin B12 Vitamin C 1000 mg 2x per day Vitamin E 600 IU	Iron 15 mg	Eggs Leafy greens Beans Lentils	Chelated iron 10 mg	
Arthritis (Osteoarthritis)	Vitamin C 1000 mg 2x per day Niacin (B3) 100 mg x 30 days Vitamin D 5-10 mcg		Fruits and vegetables	Glucosamine, chondroitin, devil's claw, fish oil, MSM, SAMe antioxidants Ginger & turmeric	Adrenal stimulants (tea, coffee, sugar, refined carbs)
Asthma	Pyridoxine (B6) Vitamin C 1000 mg 2x per day Vitamin E	Magnesium 400 mg Selenium	High Vitamin C fruits & vegetables Wheat germ Almonds Sunflower seeds	Quercetin Fish oil	
Bronchitis	Multivitamin Vitamin E 600 mg		Fruits & vegetables	Fish oil Antioxidants	Milk products Cigarettes
Cancer	Multivitamin	Selenium	Fruits & Brazil nuts	Fish oil	Saturated fats

193

ILLNESS	HELPFUL VITAMINS Look for this minimum in multivitamin	HELPFUL MINERALS Look for this minimum in multimineral	HELPFUL FOODS	SUPPLEMENTS	AVOID OR REDUCE
Cancer	Multivitamin Vitamin E 600 mg Vitamin A 10,000 IU Vitamin C 1000 mg 2x per day	Selenium 200 mcg Zinc 10 mg	Fruits & vegetables Garlic Beans	Fish oil Curcumin Ellagic acid Lignans	Saturated fats
Candidiasis	Vitamin C 1000 mg 2x per day		Grains, beans nuts & seeds		Sugar Yeast containing foods Mushrooms Fermented foods
Cataracts	Riboflavin B2 Vitamins A, C, E		Fruits and vegetables		Lycopene Salt
Chronic Fatigue	Vitamin C 1000 mg 2x per day	Zinc 15 mg	Fruits and vegetables	Carnitine, DHEA	
Colds & Flu	Vitamin C 1000 mg 2x per day	Zinc 10 mg	Fruits and vegetables Garlic Beans	Echinacea Beta carotene	Dairy products
Colitis	Vitamin C 500 mg as ascorbate		Low fiber vegetables Cooked grains	Fish oil	Alcohol Coffee Wheat
Constipation	Vitamin C 1000 mg 2x per day		Oats Prunes Flaxseeds	Fiber (soluble) Probiotics	Reduce consumption of meat & dairy products
Crohn's Disease	Vitamin C 1000 mg 2x per day		Soluble fiber found in oats, lentils beans, and fruit	Probiotics Fish oil Boswelia Curcumin L-glutamine powder 5 mg	Gluten Insoluble fiber (as in bran & whole grains)
Cystitis	Vitamin A 7500 IU	Calcium ascorbate	Fruits and vegetables	Grapefruit seed extract 10 drops 3x per day	Sugar
Depression	Vitamin C 1000 mg 2x per day Folate (Vitamin B9) Pyridoxine (B6)	Iron 15 mg Selenium 50 mcg	Chocolate Fruits and vegetables Omega 3 foods (fish, flax)	5-HTP 100 mg Fish oil SAMe	Sugar Refined carbs Reduce stimulants like coffee, tea, cola Reduce alcohol Cigarettes

ILLNESS	HELPFUL VITAMINS Look for this minimum in multivitamin	HELPFUL MINERALS Look for this minimum in multimineral	HELPFUL FOODS	SUPPLEMENTS	AVOID OR REDUCE
Diabetes	Niacin (Vitamin B3) Vitamin C 1000 mg 2x per day	Chromium 200 mcg Magnesium 400 mg Zinc 15 mg	High fiber fruits and vegetables Vinegar & lemon juice	Fiber Fish oil	Refined carbs Dried fruits
Diverticulitis	Vitamin C 1000 mg Vitamin E 600 IU		Soluble fiber found in oats, lentils, beans, & fruit	Cold pressed oil blend rich in omega-3 and 6	Insoluble fiber in bran, whole grains
Ear infection	Vitamin C 1000 mg 3x per day		Fruits and vegetables	Cat's Claw tea Antioxidants Echinacea Grapefruit seed extract 10 drops 2x per day	Dairy products Meat & eggs
Eczema	Vitamin C 1000 mg 2x per day Vitamin E 600 IU	Magnesium 300 mg Zinc 15 mg		Fish oil	Saturated fat
Fibromyalgia	Vitamin C 1000 mg 2x per day	Magnesium malate 600 mg	Fruits and vegetables	Fish oil	
Gallstones	Vitamin C 1000 mg 2x per day		Fruits and vegetables	Lecithin granules or capsules with each meal Lipase with each meal	Saturated fat
Gingivitis (gum disease)	Vitamin C 1000 mg 2x per day		Fruits and vegetables		
Gout	Pyridoxine (B6) Vitamin C 1000 mg 3x per day	Calcium 1000 mg 2x per day Magnesium 400 mg Zinc 15 mg	Fruits and vegetables		
Headache & Migraine	Niacin (B3) Riboflavin (B2)	Magnesium 300 mg Zinc 15 mg	Fruits and vegetables	Feverfew	Fermented foods (miso, tempeh, sauerkraut)
Heart disease & cardiovascular problems	Beta carotene (Vitamin A) Pyridoxine (Vitamin B6)	Calcium 1000 mg Magnesium 300 mg	Seeds & nuts Omega 3 foods (fish, flax)	Acetyl-L-Carnitine C_0Q_{10} Fish oil Garlic	Sugar Salt Saturated fats Coffee

ILLNESS	HELPFUL VITAMINS Look for this minimum in multivitamin	HELPFUL MINERALS Look for this minimum in multimineral	HELPFUL FOODS	SUPPLEMENTS	AVOID OR REDUCE
Heart disease *(continued)*	Folic acid (Vitamin B9) Vitamin C 1000 mg 2x per day Vitamin E 600 mg	Selenium			Excess alcohol
Herpes				Lysine	
Hypertension	Vitamin C 1000 mg 2x per day	Calcium 1000 mg 2x per day Magnesium 300 mg Potassium 4700 mg	Fruits and vegetables Omega 3 (fish, flax) Garlic	C_0Q_{10} Fish oil Fiber	Salt
Indigestion	Vitamin C 1000 mg 2x per day		Yogurt with probiotics Bitter greens (dandelion, watercress, citrus peel) Chamomile tea	Probiotics	Alcohol Coffee Chilis Concentrated proteins
Infections	Vitamin C 1000 mg 3x per day		Fruits and vegetables	Echinacea equiv. 10 drops 2x per day Aloe vera Grapefruit seed extract 10 drops 2x per day	Dairy products Meat Eggs
Inflammation	Pantothenic acid (B5) 500 mg Vitamin C 1000 mg 2x per day	Magnesium 300 mg Zinc 15 mg	Fruits and vegetables	L-glutamine powder 3 g per day Fish oil Anti-inflammatory herbal complex	
IBS (inflammatory bowel syndrome)	Vitamin C 500 mg 2x per day Vitamin D 5-10 mcg		Beans Lentils Fruits and vegetables	Fish oil L-glutamine powder 3 g per day Fiber	Gluten Insoluble fiber (as in bran & whole grains)
Insomnia	Pyrodoxine (Vitamin B6) Niacin (B3) B vitamins	Calcium 1000 mg per day Magnesium 300 mg	Poultry Dried apricots Peanuts Salmon Sunflower seeds Tuna	Melatonin Tryptophan	Stimulants-coffee, tea, chocolate

ILLNESS	HELPFUL VITAMINS Look for this minimum in multivitamin	HELPFUL MINERALS Look for this minimum in multimineral	HELPFUL FOODS	SUPPLEMENTS	AVOID OR REDUCE
Kidney stones	Pyrodoxine (Vitamin B6) Vitamin C 1000 mg 2x per day	Calcium 1000 mg 2x per day Magensium 300 mg		Fish oil	
Leg/Muscle Cramps		Magnesium 300 mg	Fruits and vegetables		
Lipid problems (cholesterol)	Niacin (B3) Pantothenic acid (B5) Vitamin C		Fruits and vegetables	Fiber Flaxseed	Saturated fat Processed food
Macular degeneration	Vitamin A	Zinc 15 mg	Fruits and vegetables	Lutein Bilberry Lycopene	
Neuropathy	Pyrodoxine (Vitamin B6)			Alpha lipoic acid	
Obesity	Vitamin C 1000 mg 2x per day	Chromium 200 mcg Magnesium 400 mg Zinc 15 mg	Fruits and vegetables	Fish oil Glucomannan/ konjac fiber 3 g	Refined carbs Dried fruits
Osteoporosis	Vitamin C 1000 mg 2x per day Vitamin D 5-10 mcg Vitamin K 90 mg	Boron 3-5 mg Calcium 1000 mg Magnesium 300 mg Potassium 4700 mg	Dairy products (for calcium) Leafy greens	Bone mineral complex	
PMS	Niacin (B3) 15 mg Pyrodoxine (B6) 1.3 g	Calcium 1000 mg Magnesium 300 mg Zinc 10 mg	Fish oil	Herbal complex with black cohosh or St. John's Wort	Sugar Stimulants
Prostate Problems	Vitamin C 1000 mg 2x per day Vitamin D 5-10 mcg Vitamin E 15 mg	Zinc 15 mg	Fruits and cruciferous vegetables Garlic Beans	Lycopene Saw palmetto Fish oil	
Psoriasis			Fruits and vegetables	Fish oil Topical Vitamin A cream	
Restless leg syndrome (RLS)		Magnesium 400 mg			

ILLNESS	HELPFUL VITAMINS Look for this minimum in multivitamin	HELPFUL MINERALS Look for this minimum in multimineral	HELPFUL FOODS	SUPPLEMENTS	AVOID OR REDUCE
Sinusitis	Vitamin A 7500 IU Vitamin C 1000 mg 2x per day (3x per day when infected)	Zinc 15 mg 2x per day	Fruits and vegetables Ginger/cinnamon tea	Echinacea equiv. 10 drops 2x per day Tea tree oil or Olbas oil (inhale)	Dairy products Eggs Meat
Thyroid problems	Vitamin A 7500 IU Vitamin C 1000 mg 2x per day Niacin (B3) 15 mg Pantothenic acid (B5) Vitamin D 5-10 mcg Vitamin E 15 mg	Iodine 150 mcg Manganese 2 mg Zinc 15 mg Iron 10 mg Selenium 10-15 mcg		Kelp with iodine and tyrosine 2000 mg for hypothyroidism	
Tinnitus	Niacin (B3) 15 mg Pyridoxine (B6) 1.3 g	Iron 10 mg	Vegetables	Ginko Biloba Flaxseed	Saturated fat Processed food
UTI (Urinary tract infection)	Vitamin C 1000 mg 2x per day		Cranberries Parsley		Coffee and tea Soda Spicy foods

41 Favorite Foods For Dieters

Everyone is different when it comes to dieting:
- Some people want to eat as much food as possible for their calorie allotment. Others want to eat as little as possible to shrink their stomachs.
- Some people want maximum variety to keep those few calories interesting. Others want to eat the same thing over and over, so they don't have to think about it.

What all dieters share is the difficulty of saying "No, thank you" to foods they know are familiar, satisfying, filling, and yummy. So I put together a list of some of my favorite "diet" foods, all of which are fairly low calorie, very nutritious, and highly flavorful.

Proteins

Eggs – versatile, tasty, rich in nutrients and fairly low in calories. Always good for a last minute omelet dinner; or for breakfast, fill a frittata full of vegetables and enjoy a filling taste and texture treat. Instead of buying commercial egg whites, I use one egg yolk and three whites for great scrambled eggs or omelets. Similarly, I hard boil them and use one or two yolks for a dozen deviled egg halves. And I make the filling with cottage cheese and just a bit of mayonnaise. . .tastes just as good to me.

Salmon – easy to cook—plain or fancy. Rich in protein and omega 3's. Keep a couple of filets in the freezer for a welcome weekend meal. Very satisfying and yummy.

Cottage cheese – the 2% variety has one of the best protein, fat, carbohydrate profiles of all milk products and is pretty low in calories. Chock full of calcium. Mixes well with green onions and caraway seeds for a savory treat, or with pineapple for a sweet treat. Add a bit of milk, cinnamon, and a sweetener and you'll swear it's rice pudding.

Grains

Quinoa wins my vote for the best substitute for rice, especially white rice. It is full of protein and vitamins and minerals and has a satisfying, chewy texture. Add a bit of olive oil to cold leftovers and toss in a large salad for a balanced meal.

Oatmeal wins hands down for winter breakfast and a great way to get grains for those of us who don't often eat bread or sandwiches. A fiber superstar with high amounts of both soluble and insoluble fiber, oatmeal is heart-friendly. Makes a great topping for fruit crisps, a dessert even dedicated dieters can splurge on.

Barley is so delicious in soups and stews instead of potatoes or rice. It has a unique recognizable flavor and is lower in calories and higher in nutrients that many other grains. A favorite for winter soups.

Fruits

Blueberries are the superstars of antioxidants and high in fiber. It's hard to believe they are so low in calories for something so tangy and sweet. You can eat a whole pint and barely use up any of your calorie allotment for the day. Delicious on hot or cold cereal and in whole grain muffins. Eat as many as you like. As a matter of fact, eat as much as you can of all kinds of berries. They are all superstars.

Cantaloupe – available year round, this pale orange melon is super low calorie, but rich in beta carotene. And for those who look for volume in their diet food, cantaloupe fills the bill. Fill the center with cottage cheese for a balanced lunch—they make a great combination.

Bananas – though they are a bit high in calories, bananas are so rich and satisfying, they are worth it. They pair so well with cereal in the morning and give you a good dose of potassium to balance out the sodium you might eat the rest of the day.

Vegetables

Broccoli is my all time favorite vegetable. . .steamed to perfection, it is a gorgeous green powerhouse of vitamins, minerals, antioxidants, anticarcinogens, and fiber. I never tire of broccoli's familiar flavor and satisfying crunch. It is good hot as a side dish, cold in salads, cooked or raw. On top of all that, it is one of the most calcium-rich of vegetables. Eat all you want. By the way, other members of the broccoli family, like cabbage and Brussels sprouts, are close runners-up.

Kale – I only recently learned to eat kale because I learned how to cook it from a dear friend who is a great chef. She routinely adds kale to winter soups and to steamed root vegetables. The color and texture is a great contrast to winter squash or potatoes and mixed at the last minute with assorted roasted vegetables like rutabaga, beets, and onions. Full of B vitamins and vitamin K, calcium, and antioxidants, kale is a nutrition blockbuster.

Peas – hardly anyone doesn't like peas. Not technically a vegetable, peas are legumes, like beans and lentils. Legumes are super rich in protein, vitamins and minerals, and of course fiber. Peas are great alone, in soups and stews, cold in salads, added to rice for a nutrition boost. Surprisingly, slightly overcooked peas are delicious in scrambled eggs.

Onions – I rarely eat onions all by themselves, but wouldn't this world be a lesser place without them? What they add to so many dishes, from soup to hamburgers, is immeasurable. But flavor is only part of it—along with their cousins, garlic and shallots, onions are rich in antioxidants and anticarcinogens and low in calories. Eat as much as you want.

Tomatoes-another really versatile vegetable. Tomatoes are the basis for spaghetti, pizza, soups and stews, BLTs, and in summer, all by themselves with some basil and olive oil. One of only a few plants with the powerful antioxidant lycopene, tomatoes are worth their weight in calories.

I can't talk about the best foods for dieters without mentioning that virtually any vegetable or fruit is good for dieters, because they are all such a good balance of nutrients and fiber for the calories they contain. Go easy on the starchy veggies and fruits, in favor of leafy and watery ones, and you can't go wrong. Experiment with cooking and seasoning techniques, and your diet won't seem so full of deprivation.

42 Diet Plans For Every Body Type

There is absolutely no shortage of diet plans to accomplish whatever weight control and fitness goals anyone might seek. This is good, because no single approach to eating works for everyone.

Some plans focus on one macronutrient, like carbohydrates or fats; a few restrict certain specific foods; many recommend more than the traditional 3 meals a day as a way to control hunger. A few became blockbuster best sellers, like Atkins, South Beach, The Zone Diet, and Sugar Busters. Whatever eating pattern is presented, however, the majority result in reducing the number of calories the dieter consumes.

Most diet programs provide detailed menus and some even include recipes. They rarely promote counting calories, preferring instead to define portion sizes in sample menus. But a review of the plans' menus and portion sizes indicates that most end up with approximately 1200-1500 calories per day, at least in the first and second phases, when weight loss is expected to occur. This amount of calories coincides with diet programs promoted by health and government organization like the American Heart Association and the National Institutes of Health and well-known medical centers like Mayo Clinic.

The majority of commercial diet programs present eating plans and menu suggestions that cover up to about 12 weeks. The implicit assumption is that most dieters have a modest amount of weight to lose and by the end of 12 weeks or so will be ready to transition to a maintenance plan. Rarely do any of the popular commercial plans suggest what a person with 100 or more pounds to lose should do.

TYPE OF PLAN	SAMPLE PROGRAMS	PROGRAM BASICS	SOURCE OF INFORMATION
Low Carb/ High Protein	Atkins Diet Carbohydrate Addicts' Diet Protein Power Lifeplan Sugar Busters	A low proportion of carbohydrates in the diet helps stabilize blood sugar and insulin release, which promotes fat storage in the body. Excess saturated fat is avoided by focusing on lean meats and high	Books

TYPE OF PLAN	SAMPLE PROGRAMS	PROGRAM BASICS	SOURCE OF INFORMATION
Low Carb/ High Protein *(continued)*	The Paleo Diet Scarsdale Diet Schwarzbein Principle	protein dairy and legumes. Programs usually have multiple phases, with progressively more lenient diet plans.	
High Carb/ Low Fat	Pritikin Program Ornish Life Choice Diet Hawaii Diet Low-Fat Living McDougall Program Good Calorie Diet	Mainly vegetarian, these diets are low calorie because carbohydrates and proteins have fewer calories per gram than fats. It is believed that more carbs than fats in the diet is heart healthy and avoids saturated fats.	Books
Low Calorie/ Balanced Nutrients	Dr. Sears' Zone Diet South Beach Diet Hampton's Diet The Abs Diet Get With the Program Diet Jorge Cruise Diet Mediterranean Diet Dr. Phil's Shape Up Diet	These diets aim to achieve a fairly even balance between macronutrients, believing that balance promotes efficient metabolism and modest but steady weight loss. Diet plans result in an overall lowering of calorie intake by avoiding processed foods and sugar.	Books
Portion Control	Picture Perfect Change One Eating Plan 90/10 Weight Loss Plan Volumetrics	These diet plans focus on restricting portion sizes of all foods, except those that are low in calories and high in fiber and water.	Books
Quick Weight Loss	14-Day Beauty Boot Camp Cabbage Soup Diet Grapefruit Diet Rotation Diet	Quick weight loss diets are designed to be very low calorie and very short term, usually focusing on one or two specific foods, in order to achieve rapid weight loss over a week or two.	Word of mouth Websites Books
Vegetarian	Macrobiotic Diet Raw Food Diet	Vegetarian diets are not necessarily weight loss diets, but in eliminating animal products, they tend to have lower fat and protein intake than non-vegetarians.	Books Cookbooks
Detox	Detox Diet Fat-Flush Diet	Aimed at removing all kinds of toxins and pollutants from tissues, blood,	Books

TYPE OF PLAN	SAMPLE PROGRAMS	PROGRAM BASICS	SOURCE OF INFORMATION
Detox *(continued)*	Juice Fasts Living Beauty Detox Liver Cleansing Diet	organs, and fluids of the body, including pesticides, auto emissions, carcinogens, & food-borne bacteria. Usually include a 1-3 day fast during which only water and fruit juice are consumed.	
Food Combining	Fit for Life New Beverly Hills Diet Hay Diet Somersizing	It is believed that eating certain foods in combination promotes efficient metabolism, and other combinations inhibit complete digestion, thus producing putrefaction in the intestines. Weight loss results from correct combining of food types.	Books
Body Typing	Eat Right for Your Type Body Code Metabolic Typing	The food content of one's diet should reflect what is best tolerated by the body, based on your blood type.	Books
Glycemic Index	Montignac Method Glucose Revolution Insulin Resistance Diet G. I. Diet Perricone Anti- Aging Diet	The Glycemic Index is a measure of how quickly carbohydrates are metabolized and get into the bloodstream. These diet programs base food choices on their GI score. Weight loss results when high GI foods are avoided or minimized.	Books
Online Programs	Anne Collins Diet eDiets Weight Loss Diet Biggest Loser Club	These programs are low calorie with balanced macronutrients and non-specialized food products. Advice and support is provided via online information and interactions.	Membership Subscriptions
Meal Replacement	Slim Fast Herbalife Cambridge Diet Body For Life NutriSystem	Meal replacements can be low calorie, low carb, high carb-fat, and are intended to help the dieter maintain a low calorie diet by replacing one or two meals of the day with a calorie controlled, balanced drink.	Product Representatives & websites
Weight Loss Centers	Weight Watchers Jenny Craig NutriSystem Curves	Weight loss advice, menu plans, and support are provided during group meetings, usually once a week. Most programs have weigh-ins and rewards for lost weight. Based on the belief that dieters have the most success when they are accountable to others and receive external rewards.	Information provided during meetings & in program publications

There are so many diet books on the market and virtually dozens of websites providing dieting information and assistance, and more are popping up every day. It is simply not possible to keep track of the abundance of information and advice available. Here are some resources that summarize much more information about the many diet strategies, plans, and programs that are available to the consumer:

www.everydiet.org/diet - On this website, more than 300 different diet plans are summarized.

Living the Low Carb Life, by Jonny Bowden – summarizes 14 low-carb diets and has chapters on some of the myths about low carb eating plans.

Nutrition for Life, by Lisa Hark and Darwin Deen – provides detailed descriptions and sample menus for 45 popular diets.

Diets in a Nutshell, by Mary J. Scales – reviews the specifics of 88 diets for weight loss, improving health and fitness, and disease management.

43 Prescription Drugs for Weight Control

GENERIC NAME	BRAND NAMES	HOW IT WORKS	POSSIBLE SIDE EFFECTS
Sibutramine	Meridia	Increases serotonin to increase satiety	Increase in blood pressure Dizziness, headache
Phentermine	Adipex-P, Fastin, Ionamin, Obytrim	Increases norepin-ephrine and serotonin to increase satiety	Increase in blood pressure Dizziness, headache
Bupropion	Wellbutrin Zyban	Decreases domaine reuptake	Lowers seizure threshold
Diethylpropion	Anorex, Linea, Nobesine, Prefamone, Regenon, Tepanil, Tenuate	Increases norepin-ephrine to decrease appetite	Nervousness Agitation Insomnia
Dextro-amphetamine	Dexadrine Dextostat	Release of dopamine and noradrenaline	Nervousness Agitation Insomnia tolerance
Mazindol	Mazanor Sanorex	Increases norepin-ephrine to decrease appetite	Nervousness Agitation Insomnia
Phenmetrazine/ Phendimetrazine	Bontril, Adipost, Anorex-SR, Appecon, Melfiat, Obezine, Phendiet, Plegine, Prelu-2, Statobex	Increases norepin-ephrine to decrease appetite	Nervousness Agitation Insomnia

Drugs for Other Purposes that May Cause Weight Loss

GENERIC NAME	BRAND NAMES	MAIN PURPOSE	POSSIBLE SIDE EFFECTS
Topiramate	Topomax	Anti seizure	Skin numbness Change in taste
Zonisamide	Zonagran Exegran	Anti seizure	Drowsiness Dizziness Headache Nausea
Orlistat	Xenical Alli (over the counter)	Inhibits absorption of dietary fats	Abdominal cramps Nausea Diarrhea
Glucophage	Metformin	Diabetes treatment	Dizziness Metallic taste Nausea
Exenatide	Byetta (injection)	Diabetes treatment	Nausea Bruising at injection site

44 OTC (Over-The-Counter) Supplements Used for Weight Control

Green tea extract: Cases of liver problems in people using concentrated green tea extracts have been reported.

Hydroxycitric acid: Derived from the fruit of a tree native to Southeast Asia. Health problems reported include seizures, cardiovascular disorders, liver damage, and serious muscle damage.

Chromium: A trace mineral that people can get through diet, particularly meats, whole grains, and some vegetables and fruits, but is often low in obese patients. Chromium can be depleted by eating a diet high in refined sugar and white flour products, and also by a lack of exercise. Chromium regulates blood glucose levels, decreases insulin resistance, aids in weight loss, and stabilizes the body's metabolism. Preliminary studies have shown that chromium picolinate supplementation results in a reduction of body fat and weight and an increase in lean body and muscle mass. Safe at 200 mcg per day. Side effects from higher doses can include headaches and dizziness.

Conjugated linoleic acid (CLA): Found naturally in beef and dairy products, a number of clinical studies have shown that CLA does cause a reduction in fat mass; may cause stomach upset.

Hoodia: Derived from an African plant native to the Kalahari Desert. Hoodia products typically contain other additional ingredients. Its safety is not yet known.

Chitosan: Made from the starch found in shellfish. Modified chitosan is claimed to absorb anywhere up to three to six times its weight in fat and oils, preventing absorption. These claims have been challenged by several government agencies.

Pyruvate: Produced by the body as a result of the breakdown of carbohydrate and protein from food and found naturally in foods such as cheese, wine, and red apples. No known affect on weight loss.

St. John's wort: Used mainly as an antidepressant, this herb can interact with numerous other drugs.

Aloe: Sometimes marketed as an "internal" cleanser, aloe causes a strong cathartic effect in the intestines. That can lead to mineral depletion or worse if users have pre-existing intestinal issues, such as ulcerative colitis.

Cascara: An effective laxative but ineffective weight loss agent, cascara interacts with other drugs and can throw off the body's mineral balance.

Glucomannan: Derived from a plant root, glucomannan has been banned in several countries because when exposed to liquid it swells and can result in a gastrointestinal obstruction.

Guarana: A natural stimulant, guarana can increase blood pressure.

Yerba mate: Often used in a tea, yerba mate ingestion can result in high blood pressure and overstimulation of the central nervous system. It may also be linked to esophageal cancer.

Guar gum: It is used in the food and pharmaceutical industries as a thickening agent, but taken alone, guar gum can swell on contact with liquid, potentially leading to an obstruction.

Ephedra (ma huang): Ephedra and the alkaloids, ephedrine and pseudoephedrine, are sympathetic nervous system stimulants that can cause rapid heartbeat and high blood pressure side effects. The FDA banned its sale in dietary supplements in 2004.

5-Hydroxytryptophan (5-HTP): An amino acid precursor to serotonin may be beneficial in reducing binge eating. Low levels of serotonin (an important neurotransmitter) have been linked to carbohydrate craving and may play a major role in the development of obesity. Studies have shown that 5-HTP promotes post-meal satiety (sensation of fullness) and reduced appetite. Should not be used by people taking SSRI anti-depressants.

Coenzyme Q$_{10}$ (CoQ$_{10}$): An antioxidant that boosts cellular energy production in the mitochondria, the cell's energy powerhouse. Supplementation with CoQ$_{10}$ has been reported to help promote weight loss.

Fiber Supplements (Psyllium, Pectin, Guar Gum, Chitosan): High-fiber supplements, including soluble and insoluble fiber such as pectin (fruit fiber), psyllium (natural plant fiber), guar gum (Indian cluster bean plant fiber), and chitosan (derived from shellfish chitin) may be effective for weight loss. Numerous studies suggest that fiber supplements may reduce the number of calories and fat absorbed by the body, help to control glucose and insulin effects, increase post-meal satiety (sensation of fullness), and decrease appetite.

Guggulipid (Commiphora mukul): An extract of the mukul myrrh tree (Commiphora mukul) of India has been used for centuries to treat various ailments including obesity and infections. Supplementation with guggulipid effectively lowers blood cholesterol levels and stimulates thyroid function, which may help promote weight loss.

Bladderwrack (fucus vesiculosus): A source of iodine from seaweed; may be beneficial in obese patients. Bladderwrack supplementation stimulates thyroid function, which may help promote weight loss. Since iodine toxicity problems are possible, use bladderwrack products which include the iodine content on the label.

Medium-chain triglycerides (MCTs): A special type of fat derived from coconut oil may be beneficial in obese patients. Studies have shown that the substitution of MCT products for long-chain fats may increase metabolism and help promote weight loss. Due to the possibility of ketoacidosis, diabetics and patients with liver disease should take MCTs only under the supervision of a health care professional.

For All Weight Loss Supplements:
1. Check the active ingredients to learn the mechanism of action and the likely side effects.
2. Stay within recommended doses. High doses of many ingredients can cause life-threatening side effects.
3. The liver is the most frequently affected organ and the most vulnerable to ingredients in weight loss supplements.

45 Lab Tests For Health Maintenance

Normal Reference Ranges

Definition: A reference range for a particular test or measurement, is defined as the range of values that 95% of the population falls into. It relies on the fact that for many biological phenomena, there is a predictable average distribution of values.

Influences on results: It is important to take these "normal" ranges as simply average measurements for adults, because results are influenced by many factors, such as age, gender, health status, illnesses, fasting or not fasting, exercise patterns, eating patterns, etc.

Basic Metabolic Panel [BMP]

Test	Range
Calcium	8.7 - 10.7 mg/dL
Chloride	99 - 108 mmol/L
CO_2, Total	
1 y - 15 y	20 - 28 mmol/L
15 y - adult	22 - 29 mmol/L
Creatinine	
male	0.6 - 1.3 mg/dL
female	0.5 - 1.1 mg/dL
Glucose	
fasting	60 - 109 mg/dL
nonfasting	60 - 200 mg/dL
Potassium	3.4 - 5.3 mmol/L
Sodium	137 - 147 mmol/L
Urea Nitrogen (BUN)	
1 mo - 15 y	5 - 18 mg/dL
15 y - adult	8 - 21 mg/dL

Lipid (Cholesterol/Fat) Panel

Test
Total Cholesterol
    recommended   <199
    moderate risk   200 - 239
    high risk   >240
HDL cholesterol
    major risk factor   <40
    negative risk factor   >59
LDL cholesterol
    recommended   <129
    moderate risk   130 - 159
    high risk   >159
Triglyceride
    recommended   30 - 149

Thyroid Panel

TSH   0.410 - 5.90 µIU/mL
Total T4, adult   4.9-9.5 mg/dL
T Uptake   24-32%
Free T4   0.6-1.7 mg/dL
FTI   3.9-9.5 mg/dL

Hematology Panel
(complete blood count [cbc])

WBC (th/µL)   4.0-10.0
RBC (mil/µL)
    Male   4.50-5.90
    Female   4.00-5.20
Hgb (g/dL)
    Male   13.5-17.5
    Female   12.0-16.0
Hct (%)
    Male   42-54
    Female   37-47

MCV (fl)	82-103
MCH (pg)	26-34
MCHC (gm/dL)	30-37
PLATELETS	150-399
(x103/mm3)	
RDW (%)	11.5-14.5

Other Common Tests

PROTHROMBIN TIME:	
(Average normal ý 1 second)	11.1-13.3 seconds
ACTIVATED PARTIAL	
THROMBOPLASTIN TIME:	23-33 seconds
FIBRINOGEN:	190-395 mg/dL
HEMOGLOBIN A1C :	3.9-6.2%
PLATELET COUNT:	150,000-399,000/mm3
QUANTITATIVE hCG, SERUM:	
[Males and nonpregnant females]	<5 mIU/mL

URINALYSIS STANDARD EXAM (ROUTINE URINALYSIS)

Specific Gravity	1.002-1.030
pH	5-8
Protein	<30 mg/dL
Bilirubin	negative
Urobilinogen	0.2-1 EU/dL
Glucose	negative
Ketones	negative
Occult blood	negative
Waist to Height ratio:	.5:1

Sources:

nih.gov (National Institutes of Health)
labtestsonline.org/
rush.edu/webapps/rml/RMLRangesLipid.jsp

Bibliography

There is no shortage of facts about food and nutrition available in the information marketplace. Hundreds of books and websites present descriptions of every conceivable fact about food. Search "food" or "nutrition" in any library or bookstore catalog or search engine on the Web, and you get thousands of citations. The problem is not too little information, but too much. Many books on nutrition are so large and comprehensive that it is hard to find just the information you are looking for.

Food Facts At A Glance assists the reader by presenting basic information briefly and concisely. The same is true for this list of sources. I've listed only those few books and websites that I found especially accessible and useful for finding information the average person can use. I have studied many books and checked out many websites so you don't have to, unless and until you decide you want more in-depth information. Any of the following sources would be a good place to start.

Bittman, Mark. *Food Matters; a Guide to Conscious Eating.* Simon & Schuster, Inc. 2009.

Bowden, Jonny, Ph.D., C.N.S. *The 150 Healthiest Foods on Earth.* Fair Winds Press. 2007.

Hark, Lisa, Ph.D., R.D. and Darwin Deen, M.D. *Nutrition for Life.* Dorling Kindersley (DK), 2005.

Holford, Patrick. *The New Optimum Nutrition Bible.* The Crossing Press. 2004.

Nutrition Made Incredibly Easy! Lippincott, Williams & Wilkins. 2003.

Pollan, Michel. *Food Rules; an Eater's Manual.* Penguin Books. 2009.

Pratt, Steven, M.D. and Kathy Matthews. *SuperFoods; Fourteen Foods That Will Change Your Life.* Harper Collins. 2005.

Pressman, Alan H. D.C. Ph.D., C.C.N. and Sheila Buff. *The Complete Idiot's Guide to Vitamins and Minerals. 2nd Ed.* Alpha books. 2000.

Rinzler, Carol Ann. *Nutrition for Dummies. 4th Ed.* Wiley Publishing, Inc. [no date supplied]

Scales. Mary Josephine. *Diets in a Nutshell.* Apex Publishers. 2005.

Willett, Walter C., M.D., with Patrick J. Skerrett. *Eat, Drink, and Be Healthy.* Free Press. 2001.

Wood, Frank. *Eat and Heal. 2nd Ed.* FC&A Medical Publishing. 2004.

Helpful Websites

U.S. Department of Agriculture – www.usda.gov – The first and last source of information about food, from every perspective you can imagine. Under "Food and Nutrition," there is an easy-to-use search engine where you can find comprehensive nutrient information on every food, including some prepared foods. Also, www.nutrition.gov and the Food and Nutrition Information Center – www.fnic.gov – subsets of the USDA website are wonderfully rich in food and nutrition information.

The Mayo Clinic – www.mayoclinic.com – has an abundance of brief articles on specific health and nutrition issues. Though the site does have advertisements, I found the food information comprehensive and unbiased.

Encyclopedia of Food and Culture - http://enotes.com/food-encyclopedia - has detailed articles of every aspect of food culture you can imagine, each available to be printed or downloaded as a PDF.

Acknowledgments and Thanks

This book has taken shape after a concentrated period of research and writing, during which a number of family members and good friends have been extraordinarily helpful, providing not only substantive assistance, but boundless emotional support:, Bert and Dori Reuss, Lynn Antisdel, Nancy Brennan, Dixie and Charles Cocagne, Bradley Cross, Amy Currie, Jim Gruber, Wendy and Jim House, Joanne Leonard, Esther Shannon and Haaren Miklofsky, Roxanne and Ted Moore, Ann and Don Munro, Sheryl Pearson, Jan Pogue, Lynn Stern, and Nan White. But the book has also been built on years of related research and personal experience—acknowledgements and thanks to all those who have helped along the way are too numerous to mention. Thanks to you all.

And thanks also to Paula Newcomb, the artist who designed the pages and cover, for making those endless tables so readable. Good job!

In spite of all the help, I must take full responsibility for any errors that have crept into the book. Practice makes better, but not perfect.

Index

cadmium, 33

caffeine, 166

cakes, 113, 114, 122, 132, 133

calciferol (vitamin D), 21, 26, 27

calcium, 9, 10, 11, 12, 24-31, 62, 64, 67, 68, 77, 78, 80-93, 107, 108, 109, 190-199, 201

calories, 4, 11, 13, 14, 19, 20, 21, 37, 38, 39, 40, 41, 58, 61-4, 73, 77, 88, 95, 96, 105-109, 123, 124, 125, 126, 129, 130, 132, 134, 138, 140-143, 163, 164, 165, 166, 174, 175, 182, 199, 200-204, 210

cancer, 22, 23, 26, 27, 34, 42, 43, 44, 45, 46, 56, 57, 77, 78, 80, 81, 82, 83, 84, 89, 103, 108, 184, 188, 189, 190, 193, 194

cancer-fighting (see carcinogenic), 77

candidiasis, 194

candy, 15, 115, 122, 138

cannellini beans, 95

canola oil, 52, 99, 100, 190

cantaloupe, 28, 29, 45, 55, 106, 127, 145, 189, 200

canthaxanthin, 48

capers, 115

capsaicin, 43, 44, 48, 188

capsanthin, 189

capsicum, 115

caraway, 113, 117, 199

carbinol, 49

carbohydrates, carbs, 1, 9, 10, 13, 15, 17, 18, 19, 20, 34, 39, 40, 41, 50, 51, 57, 62, 64, 67, 68, 69, 70-78, 86, 88, 92-96, 109, 121, 122, 123, 129-135, 141, 143, 171, 172, 174, 193, 194, 196, 197, 199-205, 210

carcinogenic, carcinogens, 43, 44, 45, 46, 77, 86, 88

carcinogens, 204

cardamom, 113, 117

cardiovascular, 46, 173, 174, 187, 195, 208

Carnitine Acetyl-L, 184, 192, 194, 195

carotene, beta, 22, 23, 26, 27, 43, 48, 67, 71, 76, 77, 78, 80, 81, 82, 83, 84, 85, 89, 107, 189, 194, 195, 200

carotenoids, 42, 43, 44, 45, 46, 48, 101, 187, 189

carrots, 22, 23, 42, 44, 48, 58, 106, 109, 127, 135, 145, 164, 189

cartilage, 15, 32, 33, 190, 191

cashews, 28, 29, 40, 49, 51, 86, 92, 93

casseroles, 74, 76, 78, 80, 95, 109

cassia, 117

cataracts, 26, 27, 36, 187, 189, 194

catechins, 47, 188

cauliflower, 26, 27, 42, 43, 45, 46, 49, 58, 105, 113, 145, 187

cayenne, 46, 113, 189

CBC (complete blood count), 213

CCK, 181

celery, 57, 96, 97, 105, 121, 145, 164

cells, 15, 16, 22, 23, 24, 25, 26, 27, 28, 29, 30, 31, 32, 33, 36, 42, 43, 44, 45, 50, 55, 57, 171, 173, 174, 179, 180, 181, 182, 184, 191

cellular, 43

cellulose, 57, 121

cereals, 4, 13, 15, 17, 18, 40, 41, 58, 64, 65, 68, 69, 70, 72, 74, 89, 121, 122, 126, 130, 165, 200

CFS (Chronic Fatigue Syndrome), 184, 190

chard, Swiss, 79, 80, 83, 109

cheese, 13, 14, 16, 17, 24-31, 51, 52, 54, 78, 79, 107, 109, 113, 115, 121, 122, 124, 127, 128, 130, 131, 133, 135, 138, 185

cheeseburger, 131

cherries, 42, 45, 47, 56, 106, 127, 133, 145

chervil, 113

chestnuts, 86, 92, 93, 108, 164

chicken, 22, 23, 24, 25, 28, 29, 30, 31, 32, 33, 52, 114, 116, 122, 131, 133

chickpeas, 39, 47, 95

children, adequate nutrients, 10, 13, 14, 24, 25, 27, 28, 29, 30, 31, 32, 33, 50, 52, 60, 167, 184, 192

chili, chilies, 44, 48, 79, 95, 97, 113, 117, 128, 132, 163, 196

chitin, 210

chitosan, 208, 210

chives, 47, 49, 114

chloride, sodium or potassium, 28, 29, 108, 212

chlorogenic, 44

chlorophyll, 44

chocolate, 28, 29, 32, 33, 114, 115, 117, 122, 124, 128, 132, 184, 194

cholecystokinin (CKK), 180, 181

cholesterol, 22, 23, 35, 36, 46, 50, 53, 54, 57, 64, 77, 85, 88, 89, 91, 94, 100, 103, 173, 174, 175, 176, 177, 178, 185, 188, 190, 197, 210, 213

choline, 11, 12, 21, 24, 25, 64, 67, 68, 69, 70, 71, 72, 73, 74, 75, 76, 107

chondroitin, 191, 193

chorizo, 115

chromium, 22, 23, 30, 31, 109, 195, 197, 208

cider, 115

cigarettes, 193, 194

cilantro, 114

cinnamon, 114, 117, 163, 199

circadian rhythm, 182

circulation, 188, 189

Citrulline, 184

citrus, 21, 42, 47, 196

CLA (conjugated linolenic acid), 54, 208

clementine, 106

clover, 47

cloves, 48, 114, 115, 117, 188

CMO, 191

CNS (central nervous system), 185

cobalamin (vitamin b12), 21, 24, 25, 30, 31, 193

cobalt, 30, 31

cocoa, 47, 70, 164, 165
coconuts, coconut oil, 54, 86, 87, 92, 93, 99, 100, 102, 163
coffee, 113, 138, 164, 193, 196
cohosh, black, 197
cola, 131, 194
cold, common, 28, 29, 99, 194, 195
coleslaw, 131
colitis, 60, 194
collagen, 26, 27, 36
collards, collard greens, 26, 27, 77, 78, 79, 81, 82, 121
colon, 26, 27, 43, 44, 45, 57, 188, 189
combinations, food, 141
Commiphora, 210
comparisons, nutrient, 121, 125
condiments, 124, 164
constipation, 57, 194
control,
    portion, 125, 126, 134, 166, 180, 203, 206, 207, 208
    weight, 125, 126, 134, 166, 180, 203, 206, 207, 208
Conversions, Measurement, 144
cookies, 13, 15, 16, 18, 67, 103, 113, 116
cooking, 96, 98, 99, 100, 101, 103, 113, 115, 116, 129, 137, 139, 145
copper, 9, 10, 11, 12, 30, 31
CoQ10, 210
coriander, 114, 117
corn, sweet, 9, 24, 25, 40, 44, 46, 49, 52, 53, 56, 58, 63, 64, 70, 71, 94-100, 106, 121, 122, 127, 145, 186
cornmeal, 65
cortisol, 179, 182
cortisone, 50
cottage cheese, 13, 16, 17, 24, 25, 26, 27, 28, 29, 52, 163, 185, 199, 200
Coumestrol, 47
Courmarins, 44
couscous, 114
cowbeans, 95
COX, 36
crabs, 49
crackers, 13, 15, 16, 18, 68, 97, 109
cramping, 60
cranberries, 26, 27, 35, 43, 47, 48, 62, 188, 198
cravings, 166, 210
cream, 17, 40, 79, 113, 115, 121, 122, 124, 127, 130, 132, 135, 138, 142
creamy, 86, 88
creatine, 184
creatinine, 212
crepes, 70
crocus, 116
Crohn's Disease, 60, 194

croissant, 127
cruciferous, vegetables 9, 42, 43, 47, 77, 81, 84, 197
cryptoxanthin, 48
cucumbers, 105, 121, 145
cuisine, 100
culinary, 98, 100, 101, 102
cumin, 114, 117
cup, 123, 125, 126, 127, 128, 135, 144, 96, 97, 105, 188
cupcake, 127
curcumin, 44, 48, 191, 194
cured, 114
currants, 44
curry, 113, 114, 117
Curves, 204
custards, 117, 122
cyanidin, 47
cysteine, 185, 187
cystitis, 191, 194

D

daidzein, 44, 47
dairy products, 9, 22, 23, 32, 33, 35, 86, 107, 121, 122, 124, 141, 163, 175, 185, 194, 195, 196, 197, 198, 203, 208
dandelion leaves, 35, 77, 196
dandelion, 77, 79, 81, 107
Darwin, 41, 215
deciliter, 174
Deen, Laura, 41, 205, 215
deficient, deficit, 28, 29
degeneration, 36, 45
dehydrated, 62
dehydroepian, 190
delicious, 56, 71, 74, 82, 103, 104, 107, 108, 109
dementia, 192
density, nutrient, 11, 20, 123, 134, 173, 175, 178
dental, 43
depression, 26, 27, 185, 190, 191
desserts, 72, 89, 113, 114, 132, 141, 163, 164, 167, 200, 208
detoxify, detoxifying, 45, 77, 80, 81, 107
Dexadrine, 206
Dextostat, 206
Dextro, 206
dextrose, 63
DHA, 52, 53, 186, 187, 191, 192
DHEA, 190, 194
diabetes, 3, 54, 85, 185, 187, 190, 195, 207
diabetic, 26, 27, 77, 134, 187, 210
diadzein, 190
diallyl, 49
diarrhea, 60, 63, 207
diet, 78, 94, 124, 125, 129, 133, 202, 203, 204, 205, 215

dietary, 9, 13, 15, 19, 26, 27, 32, 33, 36, 50, 54, 59, 86
dieters, 138, 166, 199, 200, 201, 202, 204
Diethylpropion, 206
dieting, 126, 163, 165, 167
digestion, digest, 4, 11, 15, 19, 22, 23, 30, 31, 36, 50, 53, 55, 57, 59, 77, 78, 79, 94, 107, 132, 134, 171, 172, 180, 186, 204
digestive, 11, 43, 171, 181, 185
dill, 47, 113, 114
dinner, 137, 140, 141, 142
dioxide, 66
dips, 79, 95, 104, 107, 114, 115, 116
disease, 24, 25, 26, 27, 34, 36, 42, 43, 44, 45, 46, 56, 59, 60, 210
dithiolthiones, 49
diuretic, 81
diverticulitis, 57, 195
dizziness, 206, 207, 208
dL (deciliter), 174, 175, 212, 213, 214
DMAE, 24, 25
DMSO, 191
DNA, 42, 43, 44
docosahexaenoic acid, 52, 186
dopamine, 185, 206
dressings, salad, etc., 16, 17, 18, 79, 101, 102, 103, 104, 113, 114, 115, 117, 122, 128
dried fruits, 58, 113, 114, 115, 116, 117, 127, 188, 195, 196, 197
drowsiness, 207
duodenum, 180, 181
durum, wheat, 67, 68

E

ear infection, 64, 71, 127, 195
eat, eating 1, 2, 4, 36, 37, 49, 54, 58, 94, 107, 109, 122-129, 137-145, 176, 179, 180, 200-204, 215, 216
Echinacea, 194, 195, 196, 198
eczema, 46, 195
edamame, 37, 39, 40, 95
eDiets, 204
eggnog, 115
eggplant, 114, 165
eggs, 9, 10, 14, 16, 17, 22-33, 34, 36, 38, 40, 46, 48, 49, 113-116, 121, 122, 124, 127, 130, 164, 175, 185, 189, 190, 193, 195, 196, 199, 201
eicosapaentenoic acid, 52, 186
electrolytes, 28, 29
ellagic acid, 44, 47, 194
empty calories, 124, 132, 141, 142
endive, 79, 82, 107
energy, 15, 16, 22, 23, 24, 25, 50, 51, 61, 123, 129, 137, 171, 173, 174, 179, 180, 184, 187, 210
Enig, Mary, 54

entrees, 4, 16, 17, 18
enzymes, 21, 24, 25, 28, 29, 31, 32, 33, 36, 42, 46, 77, 146, 171, 181, 190, 191
EPA, 52, 53, 186, 187, 191
epinephrine, 179, 185
Equal, 63
equivalents, measurement, 9, 144
escarole, 79, 82
esophagus, 46, 171
essential eutrients, 9, 10, 11, 13, 22, 23, 24, 25, 27, 33, 36, 50
esters, 48
estrogen, 42, 43, 45, 50, 81, 164, 179, 182, 190
evening primrose oil, 52
events, food and eating, 137, 138, 140, 141
Exegran, 207
Exenatide (Byetta), 207
extracts, 87, 117

F

facts, about food, 1, 2, 3, 4, 10, 12, 14, 16, 18, 20, 24, 26, 30, 32, 36, 37, 38, 40, 44, 46, 48, 52, 54, 56, 58, 60, 62, 66, 68, 70, 72, 74, 76, 78, 80, 82, 84, 86, 88, 90, 92, 96, 100, 102, 104, 106, 108, 114, 116, 122, 124, 126, 128, 130, 132, 136, 138, 142, 146, 164, 166, 172, 174, 176, 180, 182, 184, 186, 188, 190, 192, 194, 196, 198, 200, 204, 210, 212, 214, 215, 216
family, 1, 3, 49, 73, 77, 84, 217
farmers, farms, 2, 16, 17, 77, 104
farro, 68
fatigue, 184, 194
fats, 9, 10, 14-19, 20, 22, 23, 24, 25, 34, 50-54, 78, 85-99, 100-103, 121-136, 141, 143, 165, 171-176, 182, 186, 87, 193-195, 202, 203, 207, 210, 213
fatty acids, 16, 27, 34, 36, 49, 50, 53, 54, 77, 83, 85, 89, 98, 101, 103, 171, 175, 176, 183, 186, 187
fava beans, 95
fennel, 49, 114, 117
fenugreek, 117
fermented, 37, 59, 108, 109
feverfew, 195
fiber, 2, 9, 11, 34, 36, 39, 40, 41, 57, 58-96, 105, 107, 108, 109, 121, 123, 134-136, 141, 164, 172, 175, 176, 194-197, 200, 201, 203, 210
FIBRINOGEN, 214
Fibromyalgia, 195
filberts, 87, 92, 93
fish, 9, 17, 22-30, 31, 51, 113-116, 121, 122, 124, 126, 127, 141, 176, 185, 191-197
flavanones, 47
flavone, 189
flavonoids, 42, 77, 187, 188
flavonols, 47
flavor, 113, 114, 115, 116, 117, 124

flax, 48, 52, 58, 71, 85, 89, 103, 121, 194, 195, 196

flaxseed, 34, 40, 71, 92, 93, 103, 186, 194, 197, 198

flour, 64, 65, 66, 67, 68, 70, 72, 74, 86, 121, 141, 165, 208

flu, 194

fluid, 28, 29, 40, 53

fluoride, 30, 31

folate (vitamin B9), 9, 24, 25, 10, 11, 12, 64, 67, 68, 69, 70, 71, 72, 73, 74, 75, 76, 78, 80, 81, 82, 83, 87, 88, 92, 93, 94, 107, 109, 194

folic acid, 21, 24, 25, 30, 31, 62, 91, 196

frankincense, 44

fries, 114, 115, 116, 122, 131, 133

frittata, 199

fructose, 61, 62, 63

fruits, , 9, 10, 13, 15, 17, 18, 21, 26, 27, 32-35, 42-48, 56, 62, 63, 85, 86, 87, 98, 101-109, 163-166, 187, 188, 189, 193-201, 204, 208

fungi, 60

G

gallstones, gallbladder, 171, 195

gallon, gal, 144

Garam Marsala, 114, 117

garbanzo beans, 38, 39, 95

garlic, 35, 42, 43, 44, 49, 78, 79, 95, 97, 115, 117, 163, 164, 188, 193, 194, 195, 196, 197, 201

genistein, 44, 47, 190

germ, wheat, 190, 193

ghrelin, 179, 181

GI (Glycemic Index), 134, 135

ginger, 44, 46, 115, 117, 193, 198

gingivitis, 195

gingko biloba, 87, 92, 189, 198

GL (glycemic load), 134, 135

GLA, 52, 53, 186, 191

glands, 171, 179, 180, 182, 190

glucagon, 180, 181

Glucomannan, 197

Glucophage, 207

Glucosamine, 190, 191, 193

glucose, 15, 30, 31, 57, 61, 62, 63, 78, 135, 171, 181, 187, 190, 204, 208, 210, 212, 214

glucosinolates, 45, 49

glutamine, 184, 185, 187, 193, 194, 196

glutathione, 32, 33, 185, 187

gluten, 66, 67, 194, 196

Glycemic Index, 134, 135, 164, 204

glycine, 184, 185, 187

Glycitein, 47

glycosides, 189, 191

gout, 44, 195

grains, whole grains, 1, 14, 21, 64, 65, 66, 67, 68, 69, 71, 73, 74, 75, 109, 114, 117, 121, 124, 163, 164, 165, 185, 194, 195, 196, 199, 200, 208

gram, 126, 144, 203, 176, 177, 203

granola, 16

grapefruit, 24, 25, 48, 56, 106, 121, 127, 128, 136, 145, 188, 189, 194, 195, 196, 203

grapes, 42, 44, 46, 47, 48, 62, 100, 127, 146, 165, 188

grapeseed, 99, 100

greens, dark leafy, 9, 26, 27, 30-33, 36, 46, 48, 49, 77-84, 89, 95-97, 107, 114-117, 121-123, 127, 133, 146, 164, 189, 193, 196, 197

grits, 40, 65, 121

groats, 40, 64, 69, 70

GSH, 187

guacamole, 131

guar gum, 57, 210

guava, 47

guggulipid, 210

H

halibut, 176

halvah, 90

ham, 95, 96, 114

hamburger, 116, 128, 201

handful, 127

Hark, Lisa, 205

harpagophytum, 191

hazelnuts, (filberts), 26, 27, 86, 87, 92, 93, 99, 103, 176

hCG, 214

Hct (hematocrit), 213

HDL, 101, 173, 174, 175, 176, 177, 213

headache, 195, 207, 208

healthy, healthful, health, healthiest, 1, 22, 23, 28, 29, 54, 56, 59, 91, 104, 108, 123-126, 129, 136, 139, 140, 163-169, 173-178, 183, 202, 208, 212-216

heart, heart disease, 24, 25, 26, 27, 28, 29, 34, 35, 36, 43, 44, 45, 53, 56, 64, 85, 88, 89, 97, 100, 101, 103, 107, 173, 174, 176, 178, 185, 186, 187, 190, 195, 196, 200, 202, 203

heartbeat, 28, 29

helicobacter, 60

hematology, 213

hemoglobin, 30, 31, 214

hemorrhoids, 57

hemp, 52, 103

Herbalife, 204

herbs, 42, 68, 70, 79, 96, 113, 115, 116, 117, 163, 190

herpes, 185, 196

herring, 53, 107, 108, 176

hesperidin, 45, 47, 188

Hgb, 213

hickory nuts, 92, 93

histamines, 46

histidine, 184
hominy, 65
honey, 15, 17, 61, 62, 63, 121, 135
honeydew, 49, 106, 145
Hoodia, 208
hormones, hormonal, 21-33, 36, 42, 50, 53, 89, 103, 179-186, 190
horseradish, 49
hummus, 39, 90, 95, 127
hunger, hungry, 129, 136, 137, 139, 141, 180, 202
huperzine, 192
hydrogenated vegetable oils, 88, 99, 100, 101
hydroxycitric acid, 208
hydroxytryptophan, 210
hyperplasia, 87, 88
hypertension, 28, 29, 36, 85, 196
hypnosis, 166
hypothalamus, 179, 181
hypothyroidism, 198

I

IBS Irritable Bowel Syndrome), 196
ice, 4
illness, 2, 26, 27, 36
immune, immunity, 22, 23, 26, 27, 28, 29, 32-36, 43, 46, 59, 89, 100
inches, 128, 178
incretins, 181
index, glycemic, 134, 135, 178, 204
indigestible plant parts, 66, 96
indoles, 42, 43, 45, 49, 77, 78, 80-84
infants, 10, 27, 33, 184
infections, infectious, 43, 60, 100, 198, 210
inflammatory, inflammation, 32, 33, 36, 44, 46, 52-54, 60, 81, 83, 85, 89, 173, 186-188, 191, 196
ingredients, 59, 63, 65, 76, 79, 90, 97, 211
inhibitors, 36, 42
inhibits, 44, 45, 46, 54
inosital, 21, 26, 27
insoluble fiber, 57, 58, 94, 109,194-196, 200 210
insomnia, 196, 206
insulin, 54, 77, 103, 132, 179, 181, 185, 202, 204, 208, 210
intestine, intestinal, 26, 27, 57, 134, 171, 172, 175, 180, 181, 185, 204
inulin, 77, 81
invert sugar, 63
iodine, 9, 10, 11, 12, 30, 31, 198, 210
ipriflavone, 190
iridoid, 191
isoflavones, 42, 44, 190
isoleucine, 184
isoprenoids, 48
isothiocyanates, 45, 46, 49, 77, 80, 81, 82, 83, 84

J

K

kaempferol, 47
kale, 26, 27, 35, 43, 45, 46, 49, 55, 77, 78, 79, 82, 85, 106, 121, 187, 189, 201
kamut, 68
kasha, 70
kcals (calories), 19, 20, 67, 68, 69, 70, 71, 72, 73, 74, 75, 76, 92, 93, 141, 142
kefir, 59, 163
kelp, 198
ketchup, 113
ketoacidosis, 210
ketones, 214
kg (kilogram), 144, 184
kidney, 38, 39, 53, 56, 95
kidneys, 176, 185, 186, 197
kilo, 26, 27
kilogram, 144
kiwi, 48, 49, 56, 145
kohlrabi, 45, 79, 82, 108

L

lab tests online, 214
lab values, 212, 213
lactobacillus, 59
lactones, 189
lactose, 28, 29, 36, 61, 63
lamb, 54, 113, 114, 116
lasagna, 133
lauric acid, 54, 100
lavender, 117
lb (pound), 144, 184
LDL, 36, 46, 54, 89, 103, 173-177, 184, 213
lead, 33
leafy greens, dark, 9, 13, 22-33, 42, 44, 45, 48, 49, 77-83, 107, 113, 116, 121, 123, 189, 193, 197 195, 197, 201
lean meat, 9, 28, 29, 30, 31, 32, 33, 34, 121, 122
leavening, 66, 67
lecithin, 24, 25, 195
leeks, 42, 46, 49
legumes, 2, 4, 37, 38, 39, 47, 49, 58, 88, 121, 124, 201, 203
lemon, 36, 79, 97, 165, 195
lentils, 15, 16, 17, 22, 23, 34-39, 46, 47, 58, 94, 95, 9, 114, 116, 121, 193, 194, 195, 201
lentinan, 45
leptin, 179, 181

pylori, 60
pyridoxine (vitamin B6), 24, 25, 28, 29, 193,
194, 195, 197, 198
PYY, 181

Q

qt (quart), 144
quercetin, 46, 47, 83, 188, 193
quinoa, 35, 40, 64, 73, 109, 199

R

radicals, free, 26, 27, 42, 44, 46, 55, 187, 188, 189
radicchio, 79
radishes, 45, 105
raisins, 30, 31, 40, 55, 135
rapeseed, 100
raspberries, 32, 33, 44, 55, 106, 145
RBC, 213
RDA (Recommended Daily Allowance), 184,
187, 188, 189, 190
rda, 10, 11, 12, 22, 23, 24, 25, 26, 27, 28, 29, 30,
31, 32, 33
RDA, 9, 10, 11, 12, 26, 27, 33
recipes, 3, 5, 68, 97, 117
rectum, 171
regenon, 206
restless leg syndrome (RLS), 197
resveratrol, 46, 48, 188
retinol, 9, 22, 23
rhubarb, 47, 49, 70
riboflavin (vitamin B2), 9, 10, 11, 12, 22, 23, 85,
86, 90, 194, 195
rice, white, brown, wild, 26, 27, 35, 40, 49, 58,
62, 64, 66, 69, 73-76, 94, 95, 96, 97, 109, 114-
117, 121, 122, 123, 126, 135
ricotta, 13, 28, 29
Rinzler, 215
RML ranges lipid, 214
roast, 131
romaine, 49, 79, 83, 105
root veggies, 32, 3361, 62, 77, 84, 87, 108
rosemary, 47, 117
rutabaga, 49, 201
rutin, 45, 47, 188
rye, 48, 66, 74, 75, 113, 121

S

saccharin, 63
saccharomyces, 59
safflower oil, 26, 27, 52, 90, 92, 93, 101, 186
saffron, 90, 116, 117
sage, 116, 117

salad, salad greens, salad dressing, 58, 68, 69,
76, 78, 79, 80-83, 89, 90, 95, 97, 98, 101-104,
107-109, 113-117, 122, 127, 128, 131, 133, 163-165,
176, 200, 201,
salicylic, 48
salmon, 24, 25, 53, 114, 176, 196, 199
salsa, 97, 114
salt, 194-196
SAMe, 191, 193, 194
Sanorex, 206
saponins, 42, 43, 49, 109
sardines, 24, 25, 26, 27, 34, 53, 109, 176
satiety, 180, 181, 206, 210
saturated fats, oil, 50, 51, 52, 99, 141, 193, 194,
195, 197, 198
sauces, 113, 114, 115, 116, 122, 133, 163, 164, 165
sauerkraut, 59, 113, 114, 109, 195
sausages, 113, 114, 115, 116
savory, 68, 70, 113, 114, 115, 117, 199
Scarsdale Diet, 203
Schwarzbein, 203
seafood, 28-33, 113-116
seasonings, , 78, 79, 81, 82, 84, 98, 99, 101, 103,
113, 116, 117, 176
seaweed, 44, 210
secoisolariciresinol, 48
secretin, 180, 181
seeds, 46, 51, 58, 85, 87, 89, 90, 91, 93, 99, 101,
103, 104, 113-117, 121, 124, 195
selenium, 9, 10, 22, 23, 26, 27, 32, 33, 67-75, 85,
86, 91-93, 108, 187, 193-198
semolina, 67
serotonin, 185, 210, 206
servings, serving size, 1, 13, 14, 19, 20, 36, 56, 97,
114, 125-130, 134, 166, 176, 177
sesame, seeds, oil, 40, 48, 49, 50, 51, 52, 53, 58,
90, 93, 98, 99, 102, 116, 117
shallots, 49, 188, 201
shellfish, 9, 17, 210
sherbet, 122
shiitake mushrooms, 45
shrimp, 26, 27, 28, 29, 49
Sibutramine, 206
silicon, 32, 33
silymarin, 48
sinigrin, 49
sinusitis, 198
sitosterol, 49, 87, 88, 89, 91
sizes, portions or servings, 125, 126, 130, 134,
135, 141, 146
skim milk, 3
slaws, 81
snacks, 15, 16, 122, 137, 138, 141, 163, 167
soba, 70
soda, 15, 164, 198

Made in the USA
Charleston, SC
03 December 2010